Diabetes and Related Health Issues

Table of Contents

Diabetes and Related Health Issues

This book was created by me, an insulin-taking diabetic who manages diabetes on intensive insulin control regimes. I also watch my diet and exercise along with taking my blood sugars daily.

As you go through this book in more detail, you will find a great deal of information about diabetes related complications.

Whether you have type 1, type 2, or gestational diabetes, this site has a lot of information for all.

Throughout the site you'll have many recipes to choose from

I hope that this site helps anyone who has this disease and their control and management. The management of diabetes is all about tight blood sugar control so you can live a more productive and healthier life!

Your health with diabetes can be in really good control if you care for your-self and follow your diabetes care plan. This lessens the chance that you will experience many of the complications I have talked about in this book.

There are also many recipes in the last section of this book that I have shared. I hope you enjoy these and find them tasty as well as helpful in your healthy diet plan.

And lastly, **PLEASE do not take this book as medical advice!** I am not a trained medical person at all, but just someone who has gained a lot of knowledge over the years about diabetes since I have had it for many years. Always follow your physician's diabetes plan for you. You and your doctor need to work together!

Type 1 diabetes

Type 1 diabetes is what happens when the beta cells in the pancreas die and there is little or no insulin in the body. Children and teens are more frequently diagnosed with type 1 much more frequently than adults. Symptoms may not show themselves until an emergency occurs when the body can no longer handle the impact of extremely high blood sugar levels. This is when a condition called ketoacidosis occurs. The onset of type 1 diabetes can occur when the person affected might have experienced a strep throat or other brief illness which can launch an attack on the pancreas, and therefore, kills the working beta cells that produce insulin. So therefore, type 1 is known as an autoimmune disease.

My understanding is that lifestyles, and also family history play a role in this affliction. You do not catch Type 1 diabetes, as some people think, and it cannot be passed on from person to person. It has often been said that diabetes has been caused from eating sweets. This is simply not true. The body just fails to produce the hormone insulin from the pancreas that secretes insulin.

Early on, signs of type 1 may show in extreme weight loss even with eating a lot and a ravenous appetite. There is usually extreme thirst and frequent urination, sometimes with bedwetting. A simple blood sugar test by fasting determines whether type 1 is present or is in the process.

How is Type 1 managed? The first thing you should do is not panic, and teach your child with this affliction not to panic. Diabetes is very serious, but the good news is that it can be controlled with careful monitoring of the blood sugars, diet control, activity, and insulin adjustments.

Type 1 can lead to other serious complications if not treated properly. A close relationship with your doctor and healthcare team is very important when diagnosed with Type 1 or 2 diabetes.

Brittle Diabetes

What is brittle diabetes? This essentially rare type of diabetes is that type which is hard to control since the swings in blood sugar are unpredictable; ranging from extremely high to extremely low.

This problem occurs sometimes because there are other problems with the absorption of insulin by the body or else the person may have several types of hormonal disturbances present such as malfunctions of the thyroid gland. Hypothyroidism can cause hypoglycemic episodes with the blood sugars, for example.

Gastrointestinal problems are not uncommon in those with brittle diabetes. Stomach emptying, known as gastroparesis is a difficult situation when it comes to control of the blood sugar and the process of what insulin does in the body.

Stressful situations can cause upsetting swings in the blood sugar levels. Depression plays a factor as well in the stabilizing of the blood sugars in this type of diabetes. Women tend to experience this type of unstable sugars much more often than men.

The age group of diabetic people with this problem is usually between 15-35.

With this type of blood sugar control problem, your doctor needs to find the sources of problems that are behind it and work with these issues. An endocrinologist who is specialized in dealing with diabetic issues is best since this is their practicing field.

In some cases, people may need hospitalization in order to scale down the troubling issues and bring them under control. Some people may be selected to receive an islet transplant or even a pancreas transplant. While the outcome of this type of transplant holds a bright light of promise, there is a high potential of rejection, and as result, many immunosuppressive drugs will need to be taken. This venture is only recommended when all other forms of therapy are exhausted.

Type 2 diabetes is often labeled as adult onset, or I've also heard it as non-insulin dependent. It is much more common than type 1, especially in adults, though nowadays it is even being seen in some children.

When you have diabetes , what happens is that the pancreas is slowing down, but still producing some insulin. Type 2 diabetics are often known as being insulin resistant, which simply means is that the insulin does not travel correctly within the body and go where it needs to in order to lower blood sugars properly.

What happens in both types of diabetes, is that we lose our ability to make insulin, or do not utilize the insulin we make properly for sugar control. Sugar is very important in that it is the basic fuel for the cells in our bodies. We need insulin to carry sugar from the blood and into the cells.

All types of diabetes, are serious conditions and can lead to many health problems. Problems that diabetics encounter are kidney disease, heart disease, and circulatory problems, not to mention the effect it has on the eyes. It is very important that your blood sugar fluctuations are tightly controlled with good control of blood sugar levels.

What is good blood sugar control? The normal range should be between 70-98 fasting, and not above 130 after meals for anyone. A blood sugar level above 126 or more fasting is indicative of a blood sugar problem, especially when taken fasting on two different occasions.

Diabetic patients should look into multiple sources of information in order to figure out the best methods available to deal with their condition. A good doctor will know how to treat it right and give you the nutritional information you need to eat the right foods for control of your sugar levels.

Sometimes herbal preparations can help, though I personally have never sworn by them myself. See your doctor for further advice on this subject of vitamins.

Drugs for Type 2 Diabetes

Metformin, namely Glucophage,is one of the most popular drugs that doctors will prescribe for type 2 diabetes treatment. It belongs in the class of drugs referred to as biguanides. Biguanides are medications that will bring down the blood sugars by helping your body manage your insulin resistance. Glucophage also helps the liver by preventing it from producing the large amount of glucose and in turn, fat cells are more sensitized for insulin that is there.

This drug also helps with the levels of cholesterol and triglycerides, a common problem in type 2 diabetic people. This drug does not cause weight gain issues as in insulins or other diabetes pills. Another advantage is that Metformin also does not cause low blood sugar, (hypoglycemia).

The drug is taken usually in two or three doses daily, alongside meals. If you are taking the Glucophage XR, (brand name), extended release, it is needed only with supper.

The side effects of Glucophage can be upset stomach or diarrhea. These usually will disappear over time the longer you take the drug.

A potentially serious effect of the drug however, is lactic acidosis. This can be deadly if not treated quickly. Persons that have liver or kidney problems are more prone to this side effect taking Glucophage. Also, people who consume alcoholic beverages are at a risk for this problem. Early signs of lactic acidosis are:
Tiredness
Upset stomach
No appetite
Vomiting
Trouble in breathing
Muscle pains

If you are feeling any of these symptoms, seek your doctor's advice quickly.
Glucophage, which was approved in 1994 by the FDA, changed the picture of treatment for type 2 diabetes for many doctors. Since that time after this drug was developed, other drugs followed suit shortly, offering more options to doctors for treatment.

Glucophage belongs in the class of drugs referred to as biguanides. Biguanides are medications that will bring down the blood sugars by helping your body manage your insulin resistance. Glucophage also helps the liver by preventing it from producing the large amount of glucose and in turn, fat cells are more sensitized for insulin that is there.

This drug also helps with the levels of cholesterol and triglycerides, a common problem in type 2 diabetic people. This drug does not cause weight gain issues as in insulins or other diabetes pills. Another advantage is that Metformin also does not cause low blood sugar, (hypoglycemia).

The drug is taken usually in two or three doses daily, alongside meals. If you are taking the Glucophage XR, (brand name), extended release, it is needed only with supper.

The side effects of Glucophage can be upset stomach or diarrhea. These usually will disappear over time the longer you take the drug.

A potentially serious effect of the drug however, is lactic acidosis. This can be deadly if not treated quickly. Persons that have liver or kidney problems are more prone to this side effect taking Glucophage. Also, people who consume alcoholic beverages are at a risk for this problem. Early signs of lactic acidosis are:

Tiredness
Upset stomach
No appetite
Vomiting
Trouble in breathing
Muscle pains

If you are feeling any of these symptoms, seek your doctor's advice quickly. Glucophage, which was approved in 1994 by the FDA, changed the picture of treatment for type 2 diabetes for many doctors. Since that time after this drug was developed, other drugs followed suit shortly, offering more options to doctors for treatment.

Januvia is the latest oral diabetes pill that can treat type 2 diabetics. The generic name is Sitagliptin, and the drug is made by Merck & Co.

The workings of the drug:
This drug is known as DPP-4 Inhibitors. DPP-4 is actually an enzyme you have that breaks down your incretin hormones. Since Januvia is a DPP-4 inhibitor type of pill, it will make the incretin hormones slow down and increase the breakdown of hormones. Since these incretin type hormones increase, therefore your own natural insulin productions increases. The result is a glucose lowering effect. This helps the liver to more properly work with your glucose as well also.

Since those incretin hormones are the ones that respond more to high blood sugar levels, and don't respond to hypoglycemia, (low blood sugar), the chances of the sugars going low are rare.

What effects the drug should have:

This drug has been known to lower the A1C values little by little the longer it is taken. For more on A1C look at my article on this subject. The more normalized the A1C value, the less likely you will have complications from diabetes.

This drug has also been known to lower the blood sugar levels by at least 14-15 mg on average. Post meal blood sugars can decrease by as much as 49 mg or maybe as much as 55 mg.

Taking the dose:
Sitaglitapin comes in tablet forms. The usual dosage is once per day. You can take it without food or with a meal. It may upset your stomach if it is empty. So it may be best with a meal.

As with many drugs, take the pill at the same time each day and don't switch around. That way it will help you to maintain an even blood sugar level.
Also as with many drugs, **NEVER** stop taking it without the consent of your doctor. You must be under a doctor's continual care.

Your dosage of this pill will all depend on how well your diabetes is controlled. Your doctor treating you should have records of all other pills you are taking.

Side effects
The common side effects with Januvia can be:
Respiratory infections such as frequent colds
Sore throats
A headache
Interactions
Sitagliptin may aggravate kidney problems if you already have them.
Allergies, including food allergies, dyes, or preservatives might cause a problem with this drug.
Pregnant or breastfeeding do not mix well when taking Sitaglitapin.
Drug Storage
Keep the medication at normal temperature. Do not store where there is excessive heat or moisture in a room. Always keep inside airtight medicine bottle it comes in.
Strengths
This drug comes in strengths of 25, 50, or 100 mg tablets.

Medications That Can Adversely Affect Diabetes Control

Since diabetic people often have other conditions, and take other medications to control those too, these medicines can have an adverse effect on your blood sugar control, working against your diabetes regimen.

As I've talked about, your beta cells of the pancreas release insulin, which is a response to rising blood sugar levels. There are two phases to the secretion of insulin in the system. You have a rapid first phase of insulin release, and another phase which is a delayed response. These two phases depend on the potassium and calcium levels in your pancreas.

There are three major organs which have to do with insulin. The liver, in which insulin will enhance the uptake of glucose, thus preventing your liver from making new glucose. This is what the liver does to control your fasting blood sugar levels. As far as muscle and fat tissue, the actions of insulin kicks in and will prevent the flowing of glucose from these tissues to the liver. Your insulin does this by coming into action with your insulin receptor. The insulin receptor is a protein which comes from the outside of your liver to the inside of muscle and fat cells.

The types of medications that may adversely affect these actions in your body are:

Thiazide diuretics. Thiazide diuretics are frequently used to treat hypertension. They help the kidneys by blocking the reabsorption of sodium. These types of medicines raise the blood glucose because of the fact that they do affect your potassium, and potassium and insulin secretion are linked right together.

Glucocorticoids. This class of drugs have a very large effect on your carbohydrate metabolism. They are also used as an anti-inflammatory, especially in the treatment of arthritis of the rheumatoid types. These types of drugs work against insulin, not with it. They like to start the glucose production. As a result, the entry of glucose into the muscles where it needs to go is blocked off. The result? Hyperglycemia.

Beta-blockers. Many beta-blockers are used to also control hypertension. Beta-blockers can do one of two harmful things. The first is lowering blood sugar too much into hypoglycemic stages. And on the opposite side of the coin, the can prevent the release of insulin through acting with your nerve signals that link to the pancreas. This interrupts the action of your insulin working for you when it should, thus causing hyperglycemia.

Niacin. As many people know, Niacin is a drug that is used to control blood lipids, the main one cholesterol. The problem seen with Niacin in diabetic patients has been more insulin resistance. In other words, your body does not use the insulin in the correct way.

Antipsychotic drugs. These drugs have been studied as to why they either actually promote the onset of diabetes, or worsen diabetes already there. The main concept seems to be that they severely restrict insulin secretion needed in the body, and also promote a lot of weight gain which hurts diabetes control even further. They have also been known to bring on ketoacidosis in type 1 diabetics.

Every medication has some side effects, as no medicine is without this. But a knowledgeable doctor or nurse practitioner should know what to do in order to not give medications that interfere with diabetes control. A good practitioner therefore, is armed with the right knowledge to help their patients in the best way. But for you as a patient to understand the medicines you are taking, will help you and your health care team make informed decisions.

Fitness and Diabetes-

Exercise along with a good healthy diet and the right nutrition, helps decrease your body fat, which type 2's are more prone to like myself for instance. It helps to normalize the glucose metabolism, and decreases your coronary risk quite a bit. there are ways to help with your health and safety.
Another positive side to walking every day at least for 15 minutes is that it does serve to lower your high cholesterol, and helps hypertension.in athletic training, strength development, overall fitness and health

Cardiac conditioning should be the foundation of your exercise program. Try for at least 20 minutes of sustained activity three to five days a week. If you suffer from problems with your feet, skip things such as jogging or step exercises. Try instead for even strolling. This is better than no activity at all, and has some advantages.
Fluid intake is very important during physical activity when you are diabetic. If you are taking pills or insulin, then you need to consider taking a high-glucose sports drink like Gatorade or fruit juices to keep your blood sugars stabilized and from going too low. Drink your fluid before you work out to begin with,especially when taking a brisk walk as brisk walking will really lower your sugars and can make you hypoglycemic before you know it.

Flexibility exercises are important too, also referred to as stretching. This form of activity helps to keep joints flexible and reduces the chances of injury during other activities. Some nice gentle stretching for about 5-10 minutes helps your body to warm up, and prepare for walking or aerobic activity.

Exercise is a great physical therapy. It is sometimes wise to get a bit of professional guidance to begin the right program for you. You and your dietitian or doctor can work together to fit your exercise schedule into your health plan. The pay offs are great and from my own experience, helps me to maintain my weight. You can maintain your weight too with the right fitness plan.

A Fitness Partner is a Great Benefit for Motivation in Exercise and Fitness

In a quest for a healthier lifestyle, women know that fitness and exercise are important. Exercise can improve your health, increase your energy level, relieve stress, and help you to sleep better. A fit woman will remain stronger and more independent as she ages.

Sometimes the road to fitness is a difficult path when you are attempting to initiate and exercise program and eat healthier alone. Attempting to exercise daily, watching your nutrition, and making healthy lifestyle changes are often overshadowed by boredom or a too busy lifestyle. At one time or another, most women have had trouble starting or sticking with a fitness or exercise program.

Being a fit woman does not have to mean a solo journey. If you have ever had trouble initiating a fitness program or sticking with the exercise program you have started, a fitness partner may be the solution. A fitness partner is a powerful motivator. Being accountable to a fitness partner can help you start a new exercise program or stick with the exercise program over time as you continue on your road to fitness.

The right fitness partner can motivate you to achieve your fitness goals. Your fitness partner should be positive and supportive as she encourages and supports you. In choosing a fitness partner, look for someone whose fitness level is close to yours. As you become fit together, you can progress at a similar pace, and encourage each other to climb to new levels of fitness. Having similar fitness goals will allow you and your fitness partner to share triumphs and encourage you to accomplish individual fitness goals.

Keep lines of communication open with your fitness partner. A good fitness partner is honest and sensitive. Cheer each other on in your fitness successes and avoid being critical.

In addition to a fitness partner, the right fitness program is also important to achieve health. Sisters in Sneakers provides a complete home fitness program and exercise program designed especially for the fitness needs of women. Sisters in Sneakers includes color coded exercise cards for flexibility, strengthening, and cardiovascular exercises so you can vary your exercise routine day to day. Since exercise alone is not enough for a healthy lifestyle, Sisters in Sneakers includes nutritional information including fat and calorie awareness to get your eating on the right track.

Top Ten Reasons You Are Not Getting the Results You Want From Your Exercise Program

If you are not getting the results you would like from your current exercise program may be the cause is listed below.

1. Not having an identifiable goal - Most people do not pick a quantifiable measure for their success. For example "to get in better shape" - how will you know what better shape is? You need to be able to measure when you are there or better yet halfway there. Better to have something like a waist measurement goal and break that down into smaller measurements over a period of time.

2. Too many changes - Many people want fast dramatic results and attempt too many big changes at once such as a new exercise program and improved eating plan all starting in the same week. Remember you can't light a big fire.

3. Lifestyle factors - People have other factors other than their lack of exercise contributing to their current state of health. Such as not getting enough sleep, but they claim to not be able to get up an hour early to hit the gym on the way to work. Other factors that can get in the way of your health and fitness plans are stress, activity level at work, relationship stress. All of which can contribute to a lack of energy for a demanding workout.

4. Exercise selection - The majority of your effort should be spent on working multiple major muscle groups together with compound lifts. The more muscles you can train with one movement pattern the better as it burns the most calories and raises the heart rate. Additionally these exercises tire the smaller muscles so these muscles require less direct attention to reach fatigue. The idea is to raise the metabolic rate so the each exercise needs to be as challenging and interesting as possible.

5. Exercise variation - Your body adapts quickly to an exercise program and it needs to be changed every 4-6 weeks. Many people keep the same program for six months or longer and wonder why they do not see results. It is important to keep your program fresh to maximize results and enhance enjoyment.

6. Eating plan ? The results of your exercise program is directly related to the fuel you give your body. If you are not eating properly do not expect to be able to train at optimal intensity with your program. The best way to fuel your workout is with 4-6 small meals spread every 2-3 hours throughout the day. These meals should always contain 20 ? 30 grams of protein and be made up of natural, whole foods as much as possible.

7. Staying motivated - Without a clear goal it is hard to stay motivated. Setting workout related goals such as becoming stronger through increased weight or resistance or beating your number of repetitions from your last workout will keep you motivated to increase performance. Small consistent increases in performance from workout to workout will result in better results in the long term.

8. Consistency ? Changes to your eating and your exercise program need to be maintained over a long period of time to see results. Stop start type exercise will not result in progress and will only cause frustration. Don't start off trying to go to the gym 3-4 times per week. Get 1-2 times cemented into your life for a period of say 3-6 months before you add any extra sessions. You would get way better results even going to the gym once per week rather than every day for six weeks and stopping because you cannot maintain that pace.

9. Intensity and frequency -.Many people go to the gym for an hour per day, yet see no results and in most cases they are training at too low intensity (degree of difficulty) for a longer period, or more often than necessary. Doing a workout that is too low in intensity more frequently will still produce no change. You can train long or you can train hard ? but you

can't do both! Shoot for performing the most work in the shortest possible time for best results.

10 .Progressive overload ? All exercise training needs small increases or progression in workload to keep forcing your body to get stronger. Repeating the same level of intensity will cause no change to occur. These small changes add up to big results over a period of time.

Calorie burning is what creates loss of weight. Did you realize that there are many activities that burn calories that you can piece in every day? In this article, I am going to list some things that you can do in order to be on your way to calorie burning success.

The whole idea is to find ways to do activity in your daily life where you are actually burning off pounds.

One of the things you can do is park further away. When you are going to the store, the mall, post office, or any other place, make yourself walk by parking further out. If you are a bus rider, get off a few stops from your actual destination, and walk the remainder of the way.

Activity that you do at home and outdoors also counts. Look at the table below for approximate calorie burning activity that I'll bet you never even think of as burning calories:

Sleeping actually burns up to 10 calories every ten minutes.
Sitting and watching television burns up to 10 calories each ten minutes.
Dressing or bathing can take off up to 26 calories per 10 minutes duration.
Standing will likely burn 12 calories for up to 10 minutes of standing time.

Activities that are locomotion types:

Going upstairs burns 146 calories for 10 minutes duration time.

Going downstairs will burn off up to 56 calories for ten minutes duration.

Walking at 2 mph burns 29 calories approximately, and walking at least 4 mph will burn 52 calories per 10 minutes duration.

Running at 5 mph will burn off at least 90 calories at 10 minutes duration, while running at 12 mph will take off 164 calories for 10 minutes.

Cycling at 5.5 mph will burn 42 calories at 10 minutes time, or cycling at 13 mph will take off 89 calories at 10 minutes time.

Housework burns more calories than you think. The following chores burn calories:

Making your bed burns at least 32 calories if done steadily for 10 minutes.

Washing floors for at least 10 minutes burns 38 calories.

Window washing done for at least 10 minutes burns 35 calories.

Dusting for 10 minutes burns up to 22 calories each.

Cooking meals and working in the kitchen burns 32 calories for each 10 minute steady duration time.

Weeding for each 10 minutes burns about 50 calories.

Mowing grass for 10 minutes each burns 34 calories.

Activity which is recreational

Recreational activities can burn quite a few calories while doing them. The following activity burns an approximate number of calories:

Badminton burns about 43 calories in 10 minutes.

Baseball burns up to 39 calories in 10 minutes duration.

Basketball burns up to 58 calories per 10 minutes each.

Bowling nonstop for at least 10 minutes takes off up to 56 calories.

Canoeing at 4 mph takes off up to 90 calories per 10 minutes each.

Dancing moderately burns up to 35 calories in a 10 minute duration time.

Dancing vigorously takes off 48 calories in 10 minutes time each.

Football has a calorie burning rate of 69 calories for 10 minutes each duration.

Table Tennis burns about 32 calories each in 10 minutes duration.

Volleyball burns 43 calories in a 10 minute duration time.

Tennis will promote calorie burning of at least 56 calories in every 10 minutes of activity.

So activity that is continuous is what will promote calorie burning is important. This means activity without a break in between. Put it all together and you will find that your weight will change on the favorable side from doing a couple of these activities in a day.

Reasons to Exercise

Reasons to exercise number at least a dozen. I am going to list those dozen reasons here and explain what activity does for the whole body in general.

1. Sleep Doing exercise improves sleeping time since it has a strong tendency to relax your muscles.

2. Gallstone avoidance Research shows that more active women are the least likely to develop gallstones than women who are more sedentary.

3. Anxiety and Depression are relieved by aerobic activity since a walk helps to release feelings of tension and releasing chemicals which help the person feel more energetic.

4. Heart Disease Exercise boosts the supply of oxygen to the heart muscles by helping the heart muscle to expand and create tiny blood vessels. Exercise has also been known to prevent blood clots from occurring.

5. Colon Cancer Prevention is lowered with exercising. This is because the level of prostaglandins are lowered. Prostaglandins are what accelerates intestinal motility. When motility is accelerated, the movement of cancer cells speed through the colon. This is one of the best reasons to exercise.

6. Diverticular Disease Prevention risk is lowered with more activity. Why? Because walking helps to keep the pockets from the wall of the colon from becoming inflamed.

7. Arthritis pain is reduced by walking and also joint swelling goes down even with just strolling. For people that have a lot of arthritic pain, this is one of the best reasons to exercise.

8. Blood Pressure can be lowered naturally through good exercise. If you walk daily, this can definitely keep it in the normal range.

9. Diabetes Blood glucose is reduced through walking. Blood sugar levels can be reduced by as much as 30 percent or better.

10. Falls and fractures can be prevented by exercise. How? Balance training and strength training helps to prevent falls since it improves muscular strength.

11. Enlarged prostate is prevented in men who walked at least three times a week or better. There is a 25 percent lower risk of the development of prostatic hyperplasia.

12. Osteoporosis can be prevented to a large degree by doing strength training exercises. Strength training increases the bone density, and also those who take estrogen after menopause are the least likely to have bone breakage and fractures.

Foot Care and Diabetes

One of the big things in your diabetes care is to be conscious of your foot care. Your feet need to be kept free from infections, as this can lead to amputations of either all or part of the limbs. Foot ulcers are another potential problem that people with diabetes face. When you follow some simple guidelines, however, you can keep your feet free from problems.

Diabetes and Related Health Issues

Many people with diabetes have what is referred to as impaired nerve and circulatory functions. As a result, this can lead to a loss of sensation in the extremities, often the feet. When this happens, you may not feel blister, cut, or any type of sore on your foot. When you have poor circulation, it means that your blood flow to the foot is reduced, which then impacts on the resistance to infection, and leads to the loss of a toe, or even possibly worse, a whole foot or entire leg.

Half of all foot ulcer, and amputations can be avoided through care of the feet every day. Diabetics should develop a daily routine of foot care, checking for blisters, and paying special attention to in between the toes. Wash and dry your feet, and then put some moisturizer on them. This helps to keep your feet from cracking. Be careful though to not put creams between the toes, as this can cause a fungal infection.

Care of your toenails should be cut straight across, but not terribly short. Cutting toenails too short can easily lead to an ingrown toenail. File down any edges to prevent snagging. Your socks should be clean , dry, and changed frequently daily, and not too tight either. Socks that are too tight around the anklecan restrict your circulation, and this needs to be prevented.

Before putting on your shoes, you should check inside and make sure there are no obstacles inside that will harm your feet. And above all, never walk barefoot outdoors. This is dangerous to any person with high sugar levels, and can easily cause infections. In fact, this is one of the number one ways to get infections in the first place!
A podiatrist check-up is also a good idea. They can tell you how to manage your feet with your diabetes, and recommend safe products to you.

Whatever we do, we try to be comfortable. Nobody likes to be in pain. Truthfully, we do everything we can to prevent being in pain. Whether it be physical pain from an injury or emotional pain from a bad relationship, we generally seek a life without pain.

...then you get your wish and realize that you miss it.

That's exactly how millions feel who are suffering from peripheral neuropathy. Peripheral neuropathy is a condition that commonly affects people with diabetes. It can also be caused by a result of chemotherapy, alcoholism, autoimmune disorders, and a host of other conditions that we may not even know about.

So why does it happen? That answer's not so simple. Neuropathy as a complication of diabetes is caused by microvascular disease. That's the small vessels that branch of from the main pipeline arteries. The vessels stop carrying blood, which hold oxygen and nutrients, to the nerves and causes them to fail. So how do we correct this? Not easily. If that's the reason, sometimes the individual needs a procedure to restore circulation. Other times, when the main circulation is in good shape, there may be other modalities. One therapy is called MicroVas, which is a non-invasive treatment that stimulates the microvascular circulation to reverse diabetic neuropathy. It is effective based on the cause of the neuropathy. Studies have shown it to be very effective for diabetic patients, but less so for those that have neuropathy due to other reasons.

For conditions other than diabetes, the cause of neuropathy is not clear. If we don't know the cause, then it's really hard to find a solution. Sometimes the cause is a compression of the nerve, sometimes a nutritional deficiency, and sometimes for a reason that cannot be determined.

So big deal, why is this so important. Think about how you react when you touch a hot stove. Your first impulse is to pull back your hand. This is because your brain reacts to the pain even before you can feel it. And if you had no pain? You'd get a pretty nasty burn.

Now think about your feet. We jam our feet into shoes every day. What if your shoes didn't fit? The average person would take them off and figure out why. If you had no pain, you'd keep walking. What if you had a pebble in your shoe. Again, the pain would cause you to take care of it. If you were walking barefoot and stepped on a piece of glass? You see where this is going...

People with diabetes will not feel these minor injuries and can develop sores, blisters, and skin ulcers. These ulcers can become easily infected. The infection spreads to the bone and can then cause major problems. More than 60% of amputations not caused by some sort of trauma is due to complications from diabetes. This is why all people with diabetes should be familiar with a podiatrist. I routinely tell my diabetic patients that they should check their feet daily before they go to sleep and call me if they see anything that wasn't there the night before. I tell them that I'd rather they call me and it be nothing than let it go and let it develop into a problem.

The research documents that a comprehensive foot care program can reduce the rate of amputations in people with diabetes by 45%-85%. With those numbers, you should run (carefully) to your podiatrist's office. It's the first step in keeping you walking for years to come.

Footwear for diabetics is critical. Especially since it is so easy to have foot problems with diabetes. With impaired circulation problems, neuropathies which cause a loss of sensation to the feet, proper shoes are very important! Foot ulcers are born from the damage to the nerves. Then if you add poor shoes to the mix, it only makes these foot troubles more critical.

Footwear for diabetics should meet certain criteria, and not just any pair in the shoe store should be settled for.
When shopping for your shoes, keep these things in mind for good characteristics in a proper shoe:

How is the toe box of the shoe? This is the part of the shoe that covers the toe area. The toe box should be long enough to make your toes feel comfortable and not jammed inside. You should be able move your toes around. The shoe should not be too wide though, so that your feet are sliding all over the place, making falling easy. In buying footwear for diabetics, this is very important.

How about the tongue of the shoe? The tongue should be wide and padded well. You don't want the laces to dig into your feet anywhere. It is best if the tongue has two slits around the middle portion in which you can run your shoelaces. This helps to avoid slipping back and forth, and keeps the tongue right in place.
The throat of your shoe is where your foot enters. Throats should be nice and padded very well. It should not hurt your ankle or ankle bones. This is commonly referred to as the collar.

The part of the shoe that holds onto the heel is the **heel counter.** The heel is often rigid , but you should have plenty of padding to keep hard materials from hurting your feet or making them feel uncomfortable. This is another important part of your footwear.

The insole known as the sock liner is very important. When you buy a shoe with a removable liner, you can replace these that are made special to fit your foot. This insole ought to have three layers in it to provide some good wearing for the foot.

Your midsole is a cushion server for your feet. A shoe person that knows what they are talking about will know what is best for you with this shoe portion. It is the middle portion of a sole.

The arch area of a shoe is reinforced now with much plastic that is much stronger than it had been before. This is because earlier, the arch area was too flexible, causing problems with the feet placing more stress.

The outsole of a shoe is what comes in contact with the floor or ground you are walking on. Often made out carbon rubber, it needs to be very pliable and have flexibility.

Shoes with a rocker bottom will have the sole at an angle up from the floor or ground, which is at the heel and toe. This type of rocker bottom shoe helps take a load off the feet from pressure, and helps those with a joint mobility problem. This type of shoe is recommended for those with serious foot problems. Ask your doctor or podiatrist about this if you have joint problems.

Shoes you should not buy are for one, the slip-ons. Sandals are not good that have straps between the toes either. This shoe is not supportive and will only hurt your feet.

You should have your feet measured when buying shoes. Since feet tend to change over time, and with possible swelling you may have, this is why it is so important to get fitted correctly. If your feet are of the narrow type, then you need shoes that have eyelets which are wide-set. This will give you the ability to pull your shoelaces together. If your feet are wide like mine on the other hand, then you need the shoes that have closely set rows of eyelets.
When you try on shoes, bring any socks or inserts that you normally wear. This is a true test of how comfortable the shoe will really feel.
When trying on the shoes, check and make sure you feel totally comfortable with them on before buying. You should not have to break them in, or the shoe should not slide from place to place as you walk in them as I mentioned once above here. Make sure that the lacing pattern also works out best for you as well. You can often change the lacing options to suit your needs.

Footwear for diabetics then, as you can see, is a very important aspect of your diabetes management. You can never pamper your feet too much, as they are the only pair you have!

Charcot foot and diabetic foot problems go hand in hand. Bone softening occurs within the nerves of the foot and one loses the ability to feel pain or anything.Neuropathy is also a result of this complication.

Eventually the bones become weakened and will fracture easily with this condition. And because the nerves are also damaged from the neuropathy, stimuli is no longer being transmitted to let you feel pain or anything else.

When you are walking or doing activities with charcot foot, your foot or feet even, will start to change shape. Your foot arches will collapse, making you have a flat-footed shape. This is where walking becomes very difficult for you.

Charcot foot is nothing to fool around with and very serious. It often leads to a major disability, not to mention amputations of the foot or feet!

People with diabetes are prone to this foot disorder because of the fact that diabetics have strong tendencies toward neuropathies. What instigates this disorder in diabetics? Well, any trauma to the foot, going barefoot outdoors, accidents happening to the foot or feet, and any high impact activity putting more pressures on the feet. This is why it is advised to wear a good sturdy pair of supportive sneakers when walking or doing any activity. Good shoes supply extra protection.

If you come down with charcot foot, you will more than likely notice some or many of the following:

Redness that recurs or can be seen in the foot.
Swelling of your feet.
Pain which makes you have a very sore foot.
There will be joint dislocations on an xray.
Your bones become misaligned.
A strong pulse will be there in the foot.
The foot is numb suddenly and insensitive.

With any of these symptoms present, you need to get medical attention quickly. X-rays will probably be done to see your bone development.

Treatment of this problem is to stabilize the condition. Joints need to return to their original form, and therefore staying off of the foot is usually ordered.

A splint can be helpful to the foot as well. Eight weeks of wearing the splint will help further damages occurring to the foot, and you can move around without moving your foot.

If you follow the doctor's orders with proper foot care in this condition, it should cause many less problems in the end, and avoid other terrible consequences.

Nutrition and Diabetes

This is a difficult question for many. To complicate matters more, there is really no certain diet for diabetics to follow. Many people do not understand the needs of diabetes nutrition guidelines. And many people also can't understand how closely tied to good diabetic control the food you eat can be.

The American Diabetes Association has what is referred to as the Diabetic Food Pyramid. This pyramid was designed much like the old one, but provides better information on diet guidelines to help you stay in control of your blood glucose levels, and weight.

This new food pyramid is divided up into six groups. The size of the groups varies. The larger the group, the more servings per day you can consume.

The grains and starch allowances are of the largest group. This includes foods such as whole grains, pastas, breads, cereals, potatoes, corn, beans and peas. The normal number of servings per day is between 6-11. To lose weight, you should stick with the lower number of 6 servings.

The next group down is vegetables. Vegetables are naturally low in fat, of course. This makes them good food for everyone. Cabbage, cauliflower, carrots, tomatoes, lettuce, and cucumbers are examples of the vegetable group. The alloted number of servings is between 3-5 every day, though it does not hurt to go above that number.

In the middle of the pyramid is fruits. This group contains some carbs, berries, melons, apples, bananas, peaches, grapes, and others. You recommended allowance is between 2-4 servings.

Following fruits, is the milk group. This includes milk and milk products such as milk and cheeses. If you are trying for good weight control, stick with the lower fat selections in this group. The recommended allotment is between 2-3 per day.

As you near the top of the pyramid, you will notice the meat group. The meat group will include beef, turkey, fish, eggs, dried beans, peanut butter, and chicken. You only need 4-6 ounces of these foods in a day.

At the very top of the pyramid is fats, sweets, and alcohol. You should really avoid much of this group at all except for very small portions.

The best meal plan for you can be devised by a nutritionist or dietitian. The nutritional needs for a diabetic can vary from person to person according to their insulin or medication needs.

A professional dietitian or nutritional expert will be able to help you make the best of food choices while dining out, during the holiday season, and other times . And also, the nutritionist will be able to make the best of your meal plan by factoring in your likes and dislikes on many foods.

Weight loss and diabetes are very connected to one another. I am all too familiar with this scenario of staying on a diet plan-for awhile. Then after a few months or so, go back to my old ways of eating or overeating rather. I've lost weight and gained too many times to count. And some people, keep on going until they are beyond simple weight loss help. What happens from all of this overeating and yo-yo dieting is type 2 diabetes.

A lot of people start a weight loss regime, but even fewer people lose weight and keep it off forever. There are people who sometimes lose too much weight too fast. Or people will try to follow a meal plan that is far too rigid and therefore cannot stick with it for very long. The realism is that weight loss and maintaining is NOT easy! You have to retrain your thoughts toward food and your attitude toward food. Here are some pointers I have found pretty helpful:

Have Expectations that Are Livable
Is your weight loss goal realistic? Aim low, for 5 pounds. Then reward yourself, (not with food), and then shoot for the next target of 10 pounds.
What are you eating? Write it down. This is a Weight Watcher's tool and it works when you use it!

Don't look for a quick weight loss diet! Those rarely work, and you will not keep the weight off! You'll be back to your old ways in no time and have learned nothing!
Try adding in water, at least 6 glasses a day. Water does aid in your weight loss efforts and flushes out your system of impurities, etc. Another Weight Watcher's tool!

Change your food habits by the way you cook and when eating out. Another Weight Watcher tip is to go for boiled or broiled, not fried, nothing creamed, or with heavy additives like gravies, or heavy meat sauces. These contain loads of fat and cholesterol!

Do some physical activity. Walking is best and burns many calories with just 20 minutes per day. You don't have to run a marathon!
Portion control is a big one. This is one of the big keywords in weight loss!
If you are not full enough, eat raw vegetables or soups to fill up. These have very few if any calories. One of my favorite munchies is cucumbers!

Benefits of Losing Your Weight
Losing weight does carry many benefits besides looking better. You will notice less body stress on your legs and hips, and as a result have more energy. Your blood sugar may come down quite a bit, and therefore you can lower your insulin or diabetes pill requirements!

Many people that are pre-diabetic have been able to avoid the actual onset of diabetes from weight loss. If you already have type 2 diabetes, then losing even 10-20 pounds may improve your blood sugar levels.

What is your Body Mass Index?
A lot of doctors today use the BMI to measure your body fat. This gives a good estimation of your total body fat. The BMi chart compares your height and weight together. For example:
BMI
Below 18.5 Underweight
Between 18.5-24.9 Healthy Weight
Between 25-29.9 Overweight
Over 30 Obesity
Look at the BMI chart to figure out where you are at and how much weight you need to lose. Knowing this will help you to set the correct goal for your weight loss journey.

Carbohydrates:

Carbohydrates and glycemic indexes are what goes together to help you on your diabetes meal plan.

So what carbohydrates are you eating? Carbohydrates, are the term that defines starches and sugars in the foods you are consuming. Your body gets energy from this source of nutrition, but on the other hand, they have the most direct effect on your blood sugar levels. Therefore, they play the top role in your management of your diabetes.

Figuring out carbohydrates and glycemic index though, can be perplexing. It is not easy to know which kinds you can eat, and understanding how the are digested by your body. Following is what you need to know about your blood sugar, and how carbohydrates affect your sugars after you eat.

Carbohydrates are found in more foods then you realize. Many people mistakenly think they are only found in highly sugared foods. What they don't realize is that they are also found in your sources of grains and breads, milk, (yes, milk!), and even in beans and some of the vegetables have them too. Once you have swallowed these types of foods, they are quickly broken down to glucose in your blood, and raises the sugar levels pretty quickly.

To aid your glucose to move from the blood into muscle and fat cells, so it can be used for energy, the pancreas secretes insulin. In a person without diabetes, their blood produces the insulin needed no matter how many carbs they have. But with a diabetic, this is not what happens. The pancreas is either slow in producing any insulin, produces no or little insulin, or is insulin resistant. Therefore, the rise in sugars begins. And this cycle is what damages organs.

Type 2's at the beginning, will still make some insulin. But what happens is that your body can't handle a big load of carbs all at once. This is where you need meal planning. A nutritionist or dietitian can help you figure out how many carbs you are allowed. The planning is also based on many factors, including your weight, activity levels, and age. One person may be allowed 75 grams of carbs per meal, while someone else might just be allowed 50 grams. For example, one can of soup, and 2 low fat graham crackers is about 50 grams right there.

If you are a type 1, or like myself, a long standing type 2, your body makes little to no insulin at all. You then need to inject enough to cover your carbohydrate servings in a meal. If you are like myself, and set on a fixed dose or doses of insulin daily, you will need a meal plan that matches your needs. If you take mealtime insulin as a separate injection, you will need to adjust your dose to cover the amount of carbohydrate you plan to eat.

So what do you eat, or should you eat? Whole grains, beans, and starchy vegetables provide your body with the vitamins, minerals, and fibers essential to your health. Foods that are made with white flour, such as your regular pastas and any bread item that is not really a whole wheat source, have little fiber. Your fruits have vitamins and minerals, and fiber, and no cholesterol. Milk products will provide you with vitamins and minerals .

Whole milk, sour cream, and cheeses have saturated fat though, which is bad for your heart. Another good thing about carbs too, is that many of them contain a large amount of fiber, and therefore leave you feeling more satisfied at the end of a meal.

Avoid eating anything really sweet, like candy very often. They are full of refined sugars, and contain lots of just empty calories. An occasional treat of a high-sugar snack is okay, but you should exercise some caution, and not go overboard. And another side effect of this overindulging is weight gain, which does not serve well in the end.

You also need to be aware that there is a glycemic index. This index ranks foods that are carbohydrate based. Foods that have high values such as granola bars, or some cereals tend to raise your glucose levels faster than those foods with the lower glycemic values. Different carbs will affect your blood glucose differently, and with good monitoring you will know which foods have the greatest impact while others don't.

Something else to think about is fat. Fat will slow down your body's absorption of carbohydrate so that you get more of a delayed rise in your glucose.

In another article, I had touched on carbohydrates and glycemic index of foods. I wanted to elaborate further on the subject though, as this plays an important part in your healthy way of eating!

Your nutritionist should have discussed with you, how important it is to eat foods low in the glycemic index. The carbohydrates and glycemic index is simply a measurement of the effect that carbohydrates have on your blood sugar. A high carbohydrate food will break down very quickly in the bloodstream during digestion. And of course, as result, the sugars rise.

Your lower glycemic foods such as whole grains, break down slowly and therefore, the blood sugar does not rise as rapidly. Diabetic or not, low glycemic foods are a valuable healthy source to the body. Whole grains, (complex carbohydrates), give a slower rise to the blood glucose, and therefore the carbohydrates and glycemic index demonstrates this fact in your blood sugar reading which should be more stable.

Some doctor studying at a Canadian college, came upon the idea of the carbohydrates and glycemic index of food. He found that foods which were low on the scale are slower in the digestive system, and also easier on the liver.

When you eat foods with a lower glycemic rate, then chances are you will need less insulin. A food that is at least 60 or better is on the high side of this index. Many of your cereals are high in their carbohydrates and glycemic index rate, and will increase your glucose very quickly. This is yet another reason why carbohydrates and glycemic index are valuable knowledge.

You should try to eat foods that are between 55 or less. This is low in the carbohydrates and glycemic index, and has the least amount of effect on blood glucose. Most fruits and your vegetables have low ratings.

To find more information on glycemic listings of foods, I would advise anyone to look on the internet for a wealth of information available. On Amazon.com, type in "glycemic books," and you'll be surprised at the sources found there which are very helpful.

The glycemic impact diet

The glycemic impact diet is a diet and nutrition plan that is based around two core concepts, the glycemic index and glycemic load. The glycemic index is a scale from 1-100 that rates the effect a particular food has on your blood sugar level. A score of 100 is equal to straight glucose, meaning it has an extremely rapid and high effect on blood sugar. Therefore, the lower the number the slower and steadier a food's energy is utilized by your body.

Glycemic load takes the concept a bit further. Glycemic load considers the GI value, but also considers the amount and type of carbohydrates in a particular food. Some fruits and vegetables for example might have high GI values, but have a low glycemic load which means that they are very healthy to eat.

Basing around these two main principles, the Glycemic Impact diet works on reducing swings and rapid rises in your blood sugar level. It accomplishes this through a daily meal plan that is constituted of three different food groups. The first, taking up 40% of your daily calories, will be whole grains and unprocessed complex carbohydrates. All simple carbs such as refined foods, white breads and so forth have to be avoided.

Next, 30% of your calories will come from lean protein sources. The final 30% will come from healthy fat choices, those that include omega-3 fatty acids, such as avocados, nuts, olive oil and certain fish.

The foods you will be eating have low GI values and low glycemic loads. This means not only will you control your blood sugar and feel more energetic, but you'll also feel full much longer and much easier. This will allow you to naturally eat much fewer calories all throughout the day, enabling you to lose weight easily.

Diabetes and Desserts

If you sometimes or yes, often crave sweets, and have weight control issues like I do, look at these ideas here:
Try raisins, dates, or other dried fruit.

Want to eat a rich dessert? Okay, but just a small serving size instead of pigout time.
How about cutting back on the sugars and fats in your favorite sweets? Weight Watchers has some fabulous ideas for doing this. I highly recommend them for help!

Try new recipes. This makes food more interesting and it is also fun to explore.

Go for the lower calorie just as good tasting foods.

Keeping your blood sugar on target is important. To do this, you should substitute small portions of sweet foods instead of having some other high-carb containing foods combined with sweet stuff too. In other words, substitute one for the other, don't have both.

Another piece of advice is for instance, lunch. Say you are eating a bowl of soup which is fairly high in carbohydrates. You don't want to overdo it, so a good balance is one cup of soup, 4 slices healthy lunch meat, (like Healthy Choice, example), and 2 graham cracker sheets which counts as 1 carbohydrate serving. So altogether, you should only be having 2-3 servings of starch per meal. Not bad.

Check your food labels. Foods that are labeled sugar-free, low sugar, or no sugar, still do contain a lot of carbohydrate sometimes. Look at the labels for sugar content as well which tells how high the contents are in this category as well as total carbohydrates.

Be aware of sugar alcohols too. Many of your reduced calorie sweeteners have these. Sugar alcohols are mostly found in chewing gums, sugar free candies, and other carbohydrates. The ingredients Isomalt, Malitol, Mannitol, Xylitol, and Sorbitol are examples of these. There are times that these ingredients can cause diarrhea, more so with kids. Foods containing sugar alchol are not "free foods."

Your sugar alcohols do not raise blood glucose as much as other types of carbohydrates. In order to figure the amounts of other carbohydrate, you should follow some steps. For instance, subtract half of the sugar alcohol grams from the carbohydrate count.

Many people ask whether low calorie sweeteners are safe. Yes they are. They have all gone under testing to an in-depth degree before being put out there on the market. Low-calorie substitute sugars are safe for EVERYONE!

Low calorie sweeteners are an excellent alternative for adding the extra flavor or sweetness you need to enjoy your food. I enjoy desserts just as much with them as much as I do regular sugar, and in fact, find that regular-sugared sweets are too **sweet!**

Since it's based on reducing the effects of your diet on your blood sugar level, the **Glycemic Impact diet** is often implemented for people with diabetes. It's a great natural step that can be taken to help overcome this problem. It's also a great diet for anybody that's looking to lose weight in safe and healthy manner. You'll be cutting down on calories, and specifically those calories which are the worst for you.

As an added bonus, following the Glycemic Impact diet will leave you feeling more energetic all throughout the day. This is because foods high in GI value are rapidly burned through and then leave you on empty, in other words, it's the classic sugar rush and then crash effect that we are all familiar with. Eliminating as many foods as possible that do this while replacing them with low GI foods that keep you full and provide a slow, steady stream of energy will have you feeling like an entirely new person.

If you're looking for a way to control your blood sugar level naturally through dieting than the Glycemic Impact diet is a great option. Additionally, if you are trying to lose weight in a safe way or are looking to be reinvigorated all day long, than this type of meal plan will allow you to accomplish your goals.

The History of Insulin

Have you ever wondered what happened to diabetics before the creation of insulin injections? Most Type 1 diabetics before the year 1922 had to starve themselves in order to survive for any length of time. They had to follow an extremely strict diet with very limited intake on most foods, and many foods, they were not able to consume at all. Some diabetics lived for awhile, others did not survive for very long.

Knowledge about insulin is a relatively new thing.

It was a Berlin medical student, Paul Langerhans, who first discovered insulin in 1869. It was when Langerhans used a microscope , and noticed a heap of cells in the pancreas which then became known as the Islets of Langerhans. From this point later on. scientists figured out that these cells produce insulin, which in turn regulates carbohydrate metabolism. Back in January of the year 1922, Leonard Thompson, a 14-year-old diabetic,received the first injection of insulin ever. And because the extract was impure at this time, Thompson experienced a severe allergic reaction. And due to this happening, doctors cancelled future insulin injections for Thompson. In later years though, researchers were able to perfect insulin injections. This became the standard way of treating diabetes.

The concentration of insulin you inject can affect the entire body. And that explains why a diabetic person can suffer a multitude of side effects, which include blindness and slow healing wounds. People who suffer from Type 1 diabetes require insulin every day in order to keep living. Type 2 diabetics may require insulin if other diabetes pills and dietary changes are not effective enough in controlling glucose.

Right at this point and time, it is not possible to take insulin by mouth. Instead, insulin is administered through syringes with needles or insulin pens. There are some problems that are associated with insulin in treatment of diabetes. It can be difficult to determine the right dose, which often must be adjusted to meet the needs of the person. If the person taking insulin makes an accidental mistake with their dosage, it can be very dangerous.

Insulin controls the storage and release of fat, in addition to its role in metabolism. It also controls the cellular uptake of amino acids and electrolytes, and affects small vessel muscle tone.

As a whole though, when used correctly, insulin can help restore the body's metabolism to normal levels. Then as a result through proper technique of injections, people can perform at their optimal levels without any problems.

For diabetic sufferers, it is important that your insurance covers your monthly supply of insulin. Coverage for insulin use is mandated by many state laws in the U.S., and even the most affordable health insurance should cover the cost of diabetic medication.

The proper use of insulin is important for those people with type 1 diabetes. It enables them to lead a normal and productive life. Insulin will never be a cure for diabetes of either type 1 or 2. But on the bright side, research is underway to cure diabetes for good and make it a disease of the past. We may be closer to a cure than we think, but then again, it still may also be a long time in coming.

In diabetes treatment, the correct insulin dosage is important, and in fact critical Insulin is definitely classified according to how long it works in the body as well. There are five different types of insulin. They all range from short acting to the longer acting insulin treatments. Some insulins are cloudy in appearance and others are clear.

People sometimes need varying amounts of both short and long acting insulin. Every person is different and will respond differently according to their own individual needs.

There are many ways now to get insulin into your system. I plan to cover these in more detail in another article.

Rapid Acting Insulin

Rapid acting/fast onset insulin should look totally clear. It is fast acting and starts to work within one to 20 minutes. The peak action is one hour later and will last at least 3 hours and up to 5 hours. When using this type of insulin, you must eat quickly after injection times.

The three rapid acting insulins are:

NovoRapid-known as insulin Aspart
Humalog-known as Lispro
Apidta-known as Gluisine

Short Acting Insulin

Short acting insulins always look very clear. They begin to lower the blood glucose levels within half an hour. You need to have your injection half an hour before eating.

Short acting insulin has a peak effect at two to four hours, and lasts for between 6 to 8 hours duration. Short acting insulins include:

1. Actrapid 2. Humulin 3. Hypurin Neutral (bovine which is highly purified beef insulin)

4. Hypurin Neutral (this is highly purified pig insulin. It is available only via Special Access Scheme and not PBS listed.

Intermediate Acting Insulin

Intermediate acting insulins always look cloudy. They have either protamine or zinc added to delay their action. These insulins begin to work about 90 minutes after you inject, and peak at four to twelve hours and last for 16 to 24 hours.

Mixed Insulin-always looks cloudy. It contains a pre-mixed combination of either a rapid onset-fast acting or a short acting insulin and intermediate acting insulin. This makes it easier because two types of insulin can be given in one injection.

If the insulin you are using is 30/70 then it contains 30 percent of quick acting and 70 percent of intermediate acting insulin. 50/50 means 50 percent of each. You need to gently roll the vial or pen between the palms of your hands to make sure the different strengths of insulin are evenly distributed.

You need to gently roll the vial or pen between the palms of your hands to make sure the different strengths of insulin are evenly distributed.

The mixed available include:

With rapid acting insulin-NovoMix 30 (30 % rapid, 70% intermediate).

Humalog Mix 25 (25% Rapid, 75% Intermediate NPH)Humalog Mix 50 (50% Rapid, 50% Intermediate NPH)

Other Mixed insulins-Mixtard 30/70, and Mixtard 50/50. There is also Humulin 30/70

Long acting insulin

There are two kinds of long acting insulin, which have a clear appearance to them. They are:

Lantus (glargine insulin)-it has no pronounced peak action at all, which means the insulin is released into your bloodstream at a relevantly constant rate. One injection can last 24 hours.

Levemir is the other long acting insulin of choice. It also has a flat action pretty much, and can last you up to 24 hours and can be given either once or twice during the day.

These are the basic insulins on the market. They all have their unique uses for each individual with diabetes. For more about what is right for you, consult with your medical professional. This article is only given as helpful information.

The basal insulin is always being delivered over a 24-hour period and should help keep your blood sugars within your target range. So you therefore may need to adjust your doses accordingly both day and night.

Insulin pump therapy is best for those type 1 diabetics who are known to have troubles controlling their diabetes. In fact, there are even type 2's who use the pump when their blood sugars get out of control and there is no other alternative that works better. Most diabetics already realize that their main goal should be to normalize your blood sugar as much as possible. But accomplishing good control is not always that easy.

Insulin pump therapy can help you manage your diabetes control with your type of living/lifestyle. I've known many diabetics that have had an absolute miserable time trying to control their sugars with multiple daily injections and grew very very tired of keeping up with it. Especially on occasions when going out a lot! The pump has seemed to stabilize them very well.

You may wonder how insulin pumps work? Well, the pump delivers rapid or short acting insulin 24 hours a day through a catheter under the skin. You have doses which are separated into basal rates, bolus doses for carbohydrate coverage, and also corrective or supplemental doses.

Before you eat, you use the buttons on your pump to bolus insulin. The bolus amount should cover the amounts of carbohydrates you are eating. What if you ate more than you thought? Then simply program a larger bolus amount to be delivered.

A bolus can also be used to cover blood sugars which spike. Simply give yourself a correctional dosage of fast acting insulin, and this will bring your glucose back into your range.

Where do you put an insulin pump day and night? Well, most people wear it on their belt or carry a case made for the pump and attach it to your waistband. For nighttime use, you can work it so that you can clip it to your blanket, pajamas, or pillow.

When showering or bathing, you can remove the pump from yourself, disconnecting it. Most pumps are water-resistant, but still they should not be submerged into water. There are pumps that will work in a shower caddy or side of your tub.

Using insulin pump therapy is an adjustment in your daily living. But for people who have the most difficult time controlling their sugars, they have many advantages. The main advantage also being that they improve overall diabetic health, and deliver your insulin dosages more accurately. They have also been known to help diabetics with ridiculous swings in their blood sugars, and helps to stabilize more sugars into the normal range.

The disadvantages to insulin pump therapy are weight gain, and they can cause ketoacidosis if your catheter accidentally gets pulled out. They are also terribly expensive and insurances are reluctant to pay and reimburse the expenses associated with one. So these are things to think about before considering pump therapy. The pump does require some training for use as well.
To get started using a pump once you have one, your team will sit down with you and show you how to work your device, how to determine your insulin/bolus rates etc., and whether those rates will need adjusting up or down.

Hypoglycemia
Hypoglycemia is often linked with hypoglycemia, simply known as low blood sugar,and can be a very scary experience. In severe cases, seizures, or even a coma can result. Low blood sugar can result from taking too much insulin, or diabetes pills. Knowing the warning signs are very important so that you can treat it immediately!
Some of the signs you have can be the following:

You may feel fatigue or sleepiness, feeling shaky, sweating, rapid mood swings, be extremely nervous, or have confusion and not knowing what's going on.

Drops in your blood sugar can also occur when you don't eat enough food to match your medication or insulin needs. Also, after doing heavy exercise, the blood sugar usually falls rapidly, and many people have what is known as hypoglycemic unawareness. In other words, they don't realize how low their sugar has dropped until they stop exercising and nearly pass out. This has happened to me after walking several times when I almost hit the floor in sudden confusion.

Even with significant advances in diabetes treatment today, hypoglycemia is always a problem among patients who are trying to achieve better control of their blood sugar. In fact medical research has found that low blood sugar occured more commonly in patients who adhered to strict control of their sugars. Though this approach prevents complications in the longer run, these patients also had more episodes of low blood sugar.

Low blood sugar does not occur in patients who are treated just with lifestyle changes. This means that the hypoglycemic troubles are caused by too much medication. Some type 2 diabetic patients have what is called hyperinsulinemia, (too much circulating insulin). A decrease in carbohydrate intake, or problems digesting foods can cause a mismatch in insulin, and lead to hypoglycemia. Hypoglycemia is also rare in patients treated with certain drugs such as Metformin, Avandia, Actos, or other drugs in the family of sulfonylureas.

Treating hypoglycemia as quickly as possible is important at the first signs of recognition when you feel out of sorts. To correct the problem, a pack of table sugar, glucose tablets, juice, or regular soda will reverse the problems pretty quickly. Eating cake or other sweets may take too long to be absorbed into the bloodstream, thus causing blood sugars to go down even further before making a turnaround. If possible, blood sugar levels should be checked before and then again after 15-20 minutes after treating. It is also important to remember that once a the blood glucose reaches a safe level, it needs to stay at that point. It is also wise to eat a longer acting carbohydrate such as a muffin or a slice of toast to sustain the blood sugar level.

For people who run extremely high blood sugar levels, and are now getting their values normalized, may experience hypoglycemia at blood sugar levels that are actually normal. It is very important for these persons to realize that though they may feel a bit unwell, there is little chance of problems developing at these levels. Checking the blood sugar again in 20 minutes or sooner, a diabetic will know if their blood sugar is going down more, or staying in the proper range. If going down, I would eat a longer acting carbohydrate to sustain my blood sugar levels. Over the period of several days perhaps, your body will adjust to the newer normal range, and finally perceive it as being normal. **Exercise alcoholic intake with caution!**

Alcohol Consumption and Diabetes

Alcohol is a part of being sociable for many people, both diabetics, and non-diabetics alike. A lot of people enjoy a beer, glass of wine, or other beverages with a meal.

A serving of a beverage is about a 12 ounce beer, 5 ounces of wine, or else 1-1/2 ounces of distilled spirits such as gin, types of whiskey, or rum. These serving sizes contain around 100-200 calories.

These beverages are not broken down in the digestive system the way food is. The mucous lining of the stomach is the way which alcohol enters the bloodstream. From there, it will get into every cell of the body. How these beverages affect the brain is usually determined by the amount you consume, as well as by your body's metabolic rate and body composition. Moderate consumption of these beverages do have some potential health benefits. The big one for blood glucose, is that it can increase your insulin sensitivity, which in effect, will lower your blood sugars. It also lowers the risk of coronary heart disease.

On the very negative side though, diabetes and alcoholic beverages together can seriously hurt you. For one thing, when you are taking a number of oral anti-diabetic pills, strong beverages can have a serious hypoglycemic effect; lasting for many hours after words. These drinks can actually worsen some complications that you might already be having, such as a toxic effect on your nerves for instance. Neuropathy pain can increase with consumption of these beverages, not to mention other things such as eye disease, hypertension, and increasing triglyceride levels. If an alcoholic beverage has many carbohydrates in it, it can on the other hand, cause high sugar levels instead of too low. This happens in mixed drinks and sweet wines that have a higher number of sugars and carbohydrates. So beware of hypoglycemia at all times when consuming alcoholic beverages.

Depression and Diabetes

Depression with diabetic people seem to go hand and hand. I know that it has with myself and many others. It can actually be a serious complication. A diabetic with depressive issues have them on a continual or recurrent basis. And a depressed person with diabetes may not have the energy or drive to maintain good health. Depression frequently causes appetite changes, and in the diabetic youngster, suicidal thoughts. Some teens have been known to take lethal doses of insulin.

There is some thoughts I have read that psychiatric or psychological problems can affect the course of medical illnesses like diabetes. The stress of the depression itself can lead to elevated blood sugar levels, and hypertension. High anxiety levels can really affect other conditions including irritable bowel syndrome, headache, and other stomach problems. Treatment of depression definitely leads to a better medical prognosis and therefore a better quality of life.

For a number of years now, doctors have suspected a connection between the emotional patterns and course of diabetes in their patients. Physicians conducting studies have found that stressful events or other psychological illness could even precipitate type 1 or type 2 diabetes.

Since there are more accurate ways to measure blood sugars, it is easier to see both the short and long term mood factors in blood sugar levels. Children found to have more of an Type A personality had an higher blood sugar level to stress; whereas kids with a calmer disposition had a smaller blood sugar rise in response to daily stress of diabetes management.

There was a 1997 study that intimated that type 1 patients with a background of emotional illness could be at an increased risk of developing retinopathy. This group of patients were also found to have a higher level of A1C, (average blood sugars over a 3 month period). Also children whose family members played the "diabetic police," had even worse blood sugar control. Adolescents of whom are diabetic, have a much higher rate of suicidal thoughts. Those teens with suicidal ideas took very poor care of themselves.

Studies conducted recently have also strongly suggested that depression treatments can help diabetic control. Antidepressant drugs will do a lot to help diabetic people live their lives to the fullest.

A diagnosis of diabetes causes major life stresses. Diabetes requires constant care and physical accommodations. People with diabetes, kids, teens, and adults, have to learn a complex system of dietary control, and proper medical care for their condition. It consumes a lot of energy for the diabetic, and people around them. For example, my mother is my "type 3." She is the one who lives with me and hears about it on an every day basis. I know that a person has to adjust to a new outlook about their life and put it all in perspective.

A lot of diabetics will go through various stages of grief after diagnosis. There is the denial. This is more dangerous as the person with diabetes may not want to accept having it. Then there often comes anger and the "why me?", not uncommon. It may take a long time until true acceptance with being able to look diabetes in the face and go on living. I've gone through this myself as did my niece who is also a type 1. When she became a type 1 at the age of 9, her whole family was in denial at first, and it all came as such a terrible shock. I believe that with routine doctor care, every 3 months, deprssion treatment, and focusing on the positives in our lives, we as diabetics can overcome the depression factor from the disease.

Twenty Stress Reducers

Stress reducers are things you can do to release stress in your daily life and healthy ways to vent. People with diabetes tend to have a lot more stress than others since the management involves a lot of work in every day life. What with testing blood sugars often, watching diet, taking pills, exercising to keep glucose normalized is very taxing.
I came up with twenty stress reducers for people to use to help reduce their stress and even have some fun while releasing tensions. Here goes the list:

Talking to let it out is the greatest type of therapy there is. Often when you talk about your life stresses, the other person listening may have some good thoughts. This is the top of my list in these twenty stress reducers since talking solves problems many times with other people.

Start out eating breakfast. Eating your breakfast is the most important thing you can do, especially as a diabetic person. Breakfast needs to be a very healthy well-rounded meal with many nutrients to start out and especially when taking insulin.

Find Humor. Finding humor is great medicine. Read the comics, find a comedy to watch, or be around a person that makes you laugh. Studies have proven that laughing lets off stress, and therefore the stress hormone level decreases.

Find fun stuff to do. Having something to look forward to is the reason for living. In looking over twenty stress reducers, this is vital to go on living happily.

More fiber helps. How does fiber help? Fiber has been known to stabilize blood glucose, and even out the mood swings you may have. You can find fiber in fruits, vegetables, and many cereals. Diet definitely plays a role as part of the twenty stress reducers.

Eating oatmeal for breakfast is a mood uplifter. Why? Eating oatmeal helps to release serotonin from your brain which is a neurotransmitter.

Buy yourself something you like. A new book by your favorite author, or some small thing such as this helps to make a person happy and reading is relaxing, by the way.

Play with your cat or dog. Nothing is more fun than playing with your pet and brings more relaxation. I know that my cat releases stress for me since she's very eccentric, and brings me a lot of laughter and entertainment!

Stay away from negative people. Being around people that are always down in the mouth and never happy makes it harder for you to manage yourself. Stay away from people like that as much as possible. It may not always be possible, but if not, do your best to let their negativism roll off your shoulders.

Put a lid on your own inner critic. Sometimes it is easy to get down on yourself especially with diabetes. Try to tackle hardships step by step and finding solutions that work to make you happier.

Journaling helps you vent. You can write down whatever is making you very angry, why you're holding a grudge, or whatever. It is somewhere to channel grief.

Drinking certain black tea helps the neurotransmitters within the brain. The amino acids have shown to be a pick-me-up. Try drinking four cups daily.

Learn to not say yes to everything. We all have our limits, and saying yes to everything people expect may be biting off more than you can chew. Realize what your limits are in doing for others.

Having sex is often a stress releaser. There is a very large amount of endorphins released during sex that has a calming effect afterword.

Have a vacation to some place that is relaxing and get away from it all.

Board games are relaxing and fun. Try Scrabble, Monopoly, or Trivial Pursuit.

Physical activity is a great stress release for anyone. Walking helps stress hormones to go away quickly, and also gives you a chance to think.

Get a massage. Massage is wonderful and there is no better way for relaxation. I've found that after getting a massage, I can sleep much better at night for several nights after.

Take a relaxing bath. Relaxing in the tub helps a lot especially in warm water. This is because the warm water helps the body to relax a lot.

Have lunch or dinner with a friend. This is something to look forward to. A friend is also a support system.

These twenty stress reducers can be helpful to anyone, but especially those of us living with chronic health problems like diabetes. Take time each day to reflect and unwind. Life is too short anyway to be stressed out constantly, and does not do your blood sugars any favors, and in fact, will make your glucose much worse.

And lastly, an excellent website myspashop is a site with some wonderful products that can help relieve stress.

Diabetes and Glucose Monitoring

Diabetes of both types 1 and 2 require regular daily blood sugar monitoring. Testing helps you to see how stress, foods, your exercises, may affect your blood sugar levels. It helps you and your doctor monitor how well your treatment plan is working for your diabetes. At each office visit, you should take your meter in and discuss results with your doctor. From there, you can make the proper treatment plans if your current plans are not working for you.

The Diabetes Association has stated that people taking multiple insulin injections or using pump therapy, need to monitor their glucose all the more carefully. There is no suggested number of tests per day for people with type 2 diabetes, but essentially, it depends on the progress of your diabetes, and how you are treating it.

There are many blood glucose meters to choose from out there. My personal favorite is Accu-Chek Aviva or Accu-Chek Compact. I find that these meters are the most accurate and seem to match my lab results. When you choose which glucose meter you would like to use, think about what features you would benefit from on the monitor. If you like to see your trend data or past 7, 14, 21, or 30 day readings, then Accu-Chek products are really the best. People with visual impairments for example, may find that meters with a large display, or a VoiceMate meter, put out by Accu-Chek may be the best choice.

Most of your meters now read plasma glucose, while others read both plasma and whole blood glucose numbers. When you are buying your testing meter, think about the following items before you purchase it:

Size of the meter Does it fit into your purse easily to take along to a restaurant?

Time for readout How long before you will get a reading?

Memory of the meter Does it store a lot of test results? Will you get your average results?

Blood sampling size required? Does the meter require a small or larger amount of blood?

The battery life Will the battery power last a while or not? Can you easily get batteries at your local store?

Alternative site testing There are meters that allow you to test on your forearm, thigh, or palm of your hand for example. This saves the fingertips. I personally like to test on my palm!

Cost of the meter? Think about the cost when you purchase and how about the cost of test strips? Try and do this as cost-effectively as possible!

Can the meter multi-task? There are blood sugar meters that test more than blood sugar if this is important to you. One of them I know of is the Precision Xtra.

Does the meter have adaptive technology? Do you need backlighting features or not? Something to think about before purchase if this is important to you. I believe that the Accu-Chek Complete has this feature to give you an idea.

So there is a lot to consider before purchase of your meter. Consider all of the above and what you really need to have.

For most accurate testing, be sure you use alcohol swabs and wash hands thoroughly before testing. Dirty hands make for inaccurate results!

Some meters also have helpful software that you may buy with it. Both of my Accu-chek meters have Accu-chek Compass software that I have installed on my computer through their cable devices. This is really not that costly to obtain, and is a big help for me and my doctor when overviewing my current treatments every three months. I think that out of all meters, I rank Accu-Chek most highly of all. But your personal choice and needs are up to you.

The information at Health Related Fitness is helpful for anyone looking to implement a safe and effective fitness program that involves monitoring symptoms of diabetes..

Continuous Blood Glucose Monitoring

Continuous monitoring of blood glucose is a fairly recent event in controlling diabetes. It is really helpful for those diabetics who have wide blood sugar swings from extreme highs down to severe lows.

Continuous monitoring of glucose can be prescribed by your doctor. This type of monitoring system, let's people know where they are at all the time; especially in the critical stages of blood glucose swings. These types of blood sugar monitors do give you many numbers of data on graphs and charts. This is a valuable tool for helping with your daily decision making in diabetes.

As of now, there are about three Continuous monitoring glucose systems available that do provide great round figures of your blood glucose. There is the Mediatronic Guardian REAL-Time System, which you can use by itself, the DexCom Seven, that can also be used alone or integrated into a Minimed pump, and lastly, the Freestyle Navigator. The only one approved for children is the Mediatronic Guardian System.

These three systems all use a sensor which is metallic, inserted just below the skin. The sensor tracks glucose in the fluid between the cells in fatty tissue under the skin. The sensor is very thin. Devices that are loaded by springs make sensor insertion painless and quick.

The sensor records information which is carried by radio signal into a receiver or monitor. This displays a guesstimate of the current blood sugar levels. The life of the sensors used should last between 3 up to 14 days.

Both the Mediatronic and DexCom receiver monitors will provide you with updates on blood sugar readings about every 5 minutes. These monitors will also sound an alarm if the blood sugar goes way too high or too low.

Fingersticks are still important to compare readings from CGM monitoring to regular monitoring. This ensures that the CGM monitoring is accurate.
New sensors just inserted to the skin take a little time to adjust. It is often a 12-24 hour period before they become as accurate as they should.

 Fingersticks are more accurate at this time then, for a comparison sake. And since Continuous monitoring systems measure the glucose level of interstitial fluids, there is a 5-10 minute delay between the regular blood sugar meter, and the reading you are getting with CGM. For instance, the CGM monitor will probably be lower than a fingerstick done at the same time. And if the blood sugar is rapidly falling, the CGM monitor will be much higher.

The continual monitoring numbers then, should only be used for insulin dosing in the cases of the following:

Your regular blood sugar monitor matches the CGM values within 10%.
Your blood sugars are not becoming at a hypoglycemic or hyperglycemic level.
Your sensor has not received any kind of data gaps, or error display messages.

The Mediatronic device displays short-term trends within the past 20 minutes, whereas the Dexcom Seven system displays a 1 hour trend graph that has about the same information on it. The Dexcom and Mediatronic systems display three hour trend graphs. Long term trends are displayed on a 9 hours graph with the DexCom system, and the 12 hour trends on the Guardian system. The only 24 hour trend showing glucose levels is used with the Guardian integrated pump.

The best source of this type of continual monitoring is the alarm systems that will let a person know when they are too high or low. You can set your high and low target ranges on these meters, and they will give a signal if your blood glucose is off-kilter either way.

All in all, wearing a monitor which is continuous is best for someone who has more critical rises and falls as I mentioned in the first part of my article.

Hemoglobin A1C

Hemoglobin A1C. What is it and why is this test every 3 months important with diabetics of **all types ?** I am writing this article to explain the test, and why it is critical for all diabetics to have this component of their blood measured?

Your blood sugar testing that you do at home every day is important as a part of your diabetes control plan. The goal for all diabetics is to keep their sugars from 70-120 as much as possible before meals, and no more than 140 2 hours after a meal. Your blood sugar meter should make as close to accurate assessments as possible. Your daily blood sugar tests give you clues as to how to plan your meals and make adjustments with your doctor day in and day out.
Blood sugar however, fluctuates widely a lot of times that your are not aware of. This is where the reading of the hemoglobin A1C comes in.

What is hemoglobin A1C? Simply put, think of sugar that is sticking. When it sticks for a long time, it is more difficult to get it off. In the diabetic's body, glucose sticks too, especially in proteins. The red blood cells will circulate in your body on an average of 3 months before they die. When glucose ticks around on these cells, it gives an estimate of how much sugar is hanging around for the past 3 month period. Labs are all different in their methods of performing this test, but the average normal rate is 4.5 to 5.9. If a person with diabetes is having poorly controlled sugar levels, then this level is well above range from 6.0 or much higher.

There is a definite pattern between A1C levels and average blood sugar levels.

An A1C of 5 percent usually means your average blood sugar is around 125; a percentage of 6 puts you around the 135 target; with a 7 percent level of A1C or more, you're averaging out at least 170 or better, which is too high and needs to be brought under control.

It is recommended by ADA that you keep your percentage of A1C below 7 to avoid complications. Many diabetic studies have shown that an A1C kept as close to normal as possible avoid serious complications. In other words, the higher the percentage number, the greater risk for many problems related to diabetes.

The doctor being diligent about performing the A1C is helping their patients by motivating them to stick with their care plan as carefully as possible to avoid terrible medical problems in the end related to diabetes.

Diabetic Retinopathy

The retina is the main source of our vision, which actually transmits signals to the optic nerve, allowing our visual field to come through.

When you have diabetic retinopathy, the small blood vessels in the retina become swollen, and often leak fluid. There is hemorrhaging and the vision then becomes blocked. This whole process can cause an overgrowth of the new blood vessels, which are very tiny, to gain scar tissue. The separation of the retina occurs from where it is attached to the inside of the eye, causing visual loss.

Retinopathy in a diabetic is the leading cause then, of blindness. Anyone with diabetes, type 1 or 2, should have regular eye check-ups to help recognize this condition at the onset.

Retinopathy affects anyone who has had diabetes long term, (5 years or better). The risk of developing this diabetic complication and the rate of which it progresses, can be greatly reduced by good blood sugar control.

Some of the things a good eye doctor may find on examination of the eyes are microaneurysms. They appear as tiny red spots in the light-sensitive retina, right at the back of the eye. The eye doctor will also recognize some tiny hemorrhages. There is also something called hard exudates. These are one of the main characteristics of retinopathy and they can vary in size from tiny specks, to large patches. There are also soft exudates. Soft exudates are often called cotton wool spots, and are seen in the more advanced retinopathy.

In the early stages of retinopathy, there are no symptoms. But as retinopathy progresses, you will experience great visual impairments, which includes distorted or patchy vision that your prescription glasses will not help.
Laser therapy is most commonly used in the treatment of diabetic retinopathy. It is referred to as panretinal laser photocoagulation. This procedure is normally done under a local anesthetic. In this form of laser-type treatment, there are bursts of a laser beam directed toward the retina of the eye, and this helps to stop growth of abnormal blood vessels , and cut the risk of bleeding. Therefore, then it is hoped that it will reduce the risk of severe visual loss significantly. The procedure will not correct advanced vision loss.
This is why it is important to keep your blood sugar under control as well as your blood pressure, if hypertension is also a problem. Keeping your sugars stabilized will help prevent the onset of retinopathy from happening, and help you to maintain normal eye health care. Companies like www.visiondirect.com make it convenient to order your contacts but make sure if you have any of the symptoms described above to call your doctor immediately.

Protecting your eyesight is a MUST with diabetes!

Glaucoma and Diabetes

Glaucoma itself is actually classified as a group of several eye diseases that are very damaging to your optic nerve. **Optic nerves** are nerve fibers in a bundle that are the transporters from your eye to the brain. When the optic nerve becomes damaged, then this is what leads to visual impairment, and even blindness.

You need to understand first that this eye disease is in several forms. The two main forms are: **open angle,** the more common that affects more individuals than **closed angle.** The open angle glaucoma usually does not presnt any symptoms. What is lost in this case is your peripheral vision. As it silently goes on without any treatment, the visual field is gradually lost.

Now with **closed angle** glaucoma, this is usually in the form of acute, or chronic. If you are having the acute phase of this eye disease, the flow that normally occurs from the iris and the lens is blocked off. You can have a symptomatology of:

Severe pain
nausea and vomiting
blurry vision
and a halo of a rainbow type that will come up around lights

If you are having this acute type, you need medical attention right away.
In closed angle types of this eye disease, this is a slow progression, and is sneaky since it slowly takes away vision without any warnings.
There are many other forms of this eye disease such as the following: juvenile, secondary forms, normal tension, and then there is congenital. If you have the secondary type, it can either be closed or open angle, and usually is from another medical problem you have had in the body or eyes themselves.

Detecting this eye problem:

Eye doctors will give you tests in several forms and ways to find out if you have this eye condition. There is:

A visual acuity test
Visual field test for peripheral vision
Dilated eye exams to look back into the eye
Pachymetry, tonometry, ophthalmoscopy along with nerve imaging

Treatment by doctors

Treatment can be given in eye drops, pills, or both. Medications such as **Beta-blockers** will help to lower the eye pressure. It decreases the fluid is flowing into the eye. Medications such as **miotics** will help the eye with the drainage of fluid, increasing the rate so it relieves eye pressure.

Eye drops in the form of carbonic anhydrase inhibitors will help causes of lowering fluid production within the eye.

Other treatments:

Filtration surgery is used as a treatment that is a last resort when other measures fail. Trabeculectomy can be done under a local anesthetic. This procedure creates an opening so that the fluid is able to flow well and enter the bloodstream. One eye at a time is done, and an overnight stay in the hospital is sometimes needed.

Laser surgery can be useful. This surgery using a laser technique, opens the eye through trabecular meshwork, which opens visual fields.

Polycystic Ovarian Syndrome

Polycystic Ovarian Syndrome, (known as the Stein-Levanthal Syndrome), is classified as a hormonal imbalance. These women who show a high testosterone level, along with high circulating insulin, (hyperinsulinemia), have a definitive diagnosis of Polycystic Ovarian Syndrome. Infertility , weight gain, and type 2 diabetes develop along the way as well. This is actually in my case, what caused my diabetes to begin with. Doctors and researchers say that over 50% of women or teen girls with Polycystic Ovarian Syndrome contract Type 2 diabetes before they are 40 years of age. Polycystic ovaries therefore, presents a danger to young women in their late teens and older. This is why it should be diagnosed early on.

So what is it that causes some women to have Polycystic Ovarian Syndrome? PCOS first of all, means there are multiple cysts on each ovary. The cysts begin in follicles which should be producing eggs for reproduction. Because there are a higher level of male hormones, these follicles do not fully mature and instead remain as a cyst, Now since the follicles do not mature, the ovaries then produce less progesterone. Progesterone is what women need for ovulation, and so these girls and women are less like to have any regular menstrual cycles. And because there is also less estrogen then there should be, the testosterone secretions increase, and the result is PCOS.

The cysts that are developed are testosterone sources. This interferes with a woman's natural estrogen level and leads to yet more problems. The symptoms that will come up are, excess facial hairs or body hair, obesity, and periods do not come often if at all. Acne is another symptom that can present itself as well as loss or thinning of hair.

Sometimes in the more advanced cases of PCOS, patches of brown spots at the breasts, elbows, and other places on the body are present.

Many women with PCOS are also at risk for developing heart and other types of circulatory diseases. High insulin levels are harmful to a young girl's or woman's health. This causes the blood vessels to constrict, and very often leads to insulin-dependent diabetes.

What is the best way of treating PCOS? There really is no perfect treatment for this disorder. Every person is uniquely different and can be treated in different ways. Women can be given steroids to treat this disorder if the symptoms prove to be severe. In my particular case, I was treated for all of the problems stemming from this complex disorder.

Some doctors may prescribe birth control pills in order to achieve some regularity with menstrual cycles. Sometimes the birth control methods will also take care of the high testosterone levels. If type 2 diabetes becomes present, which is usually the case, then a doctor should prescribe anti-diabetes pills to reduce the effects of higher levels of insulin circulating in the bloodstream.

PCOS is a very complex female disorder then. Follow-up with a doctor is very important if you have this disease in order to try and maintain the best health possible.

Diabetes and Celiac Disease

Celiac Disease is common in people that have Type 1 diabetes. This disease, like type 1 diabetes, is also an autoimmune disorder. So then a person with the autoimmune disorder of type 1 diabetes, is then likely to have this difficult digestive disorder.

What's this about "Gluten-Free?"

The term "gluten-free" has become more familiar to American consumers than it was a decade ago. While people suffering from celiac disease once had to maintain very prohibitive diets to control their condition, manufacturers have responded to consumer needs by producing a wider variety of gluten-free products. Some of the most common gluten-containing foods that aggravate celiac symptoms include wheat, oats, rye and barley. Although the cause of celiac remains unknown, those who suffer from this disease often experience malnutrition since celiac prevents the body from properly absorbing essential vitamins and minerals.

Resulting vitamin deficiencies contribute to a variety of unpleasant disorders and symptoms. A few of these health issues include thyroid disease, type 1 diabetes, infertility, autoimmune dysfunction, intestinal lymphomas and cancers, nosebleeds, abdominal discomfort and bloating, depression, easy bruising, nosebleeds, bowel and weight changes, and oral ulcers. Symptoms and other health conditions vary from patient to patient. To diagnose patients with celiac, doctors first look for abnormal blood test results and then typically order an upper endoscopy and biopsy to determine if the disease is present.
If the biopsy indicates celiac, the doctor's primary prescription will be dietary changes. By following a gluten-free diet, most sufferers can control or alleviate their symptoms and most related conditions. When attempting to eat gluten-free, some patients discover that gluten can hide in the most unusual places. Even some fruit juices can contain additives that contain gluten or that otherwise aggravate celiac symptoms. In the past, patients had to determine by trial and error which beverages would aggravate symptoms.

Patients with celiac no longer have to do their grocery shopping exclusively at specialty stores. Even mass merchandisers carry gluten-free products. First came sugar-free and fat-free. Now, gluten-free is just "one of the crowd" at the local grocery store.

There is also "silent Celiac disease. This group of people are asymptomatic. This form is only diagnosed when the bowel is examined or biopsied because of another problem a person is having.

Otherwise the diagnosis of Celiac starts with blood testing which will search for a certain type of antibodies that are usually found in people with Celiac. If you do have these antibodies, then your doctor will need to do a series of biopsies to remove tissue samples of your small intestine. What they are looking for there is a change in tissue. This testing is done by using a special scope through the mouth leading into the small intestine.

The next step in diagnosis is to have you try a gluten-free diet for about a week or so. If you feel much more comfortable, then this is an indicator of Celiac disease present.

The key to treating Celiac disease, is to give up gluten-containing foods. I would advise anyone with this problem to sit down with a nutritional expert, or dietitian, and figure out how you can eat well, still enjoy many foods, but without gluten present.

Neuropathy Issues with Diabetes

Neuropathy can be a serious complication of diabetes.

There are types of neuropathy that I will explain here for your better understanding of it.

Neuropathy defined is damage to the nerves that make you feel the sensations such as pain, hot, or cold. Diabetes damages the nerves in a number of ways; but the main reason is blood glucose that is too high for sustained periods of time. Neuropathy can be painful, but not beyond tolerance painful. There are four types of diabetic neuropathy.

Peripheral Neuropathy

The feet and legs are most affected in peripheral neuropathy. The nerve damages in your feet or legs result in losses of sensations, increasing your risk of more foot problems. Sores, injuries, and ulcers on the feet may not even been noticed due to lack of feelings. This is why it is important to practice good thorough foot care as I mentioned in another article here. Something that is not all that common but may happen is lack of sensations in the arms, abdomen, and back.

Common symptoms of neuropathy are: **tingling, numbness, of which may be severe or long-term, burning sensations, and also pain.**

When your blood sugar is under control, you can avoid this problem. There are other preventive measures you can take such as examining your feet and legs on a daily basis, applying lotion helps if your feet are dry, care for your nails regularly, and you should also wear properly fitting shoes and other footwear to avoid injuries to your feet and legs.

Diabetic Proximal Neuropathy does cause pain usually on one side or the other of the thighs, hips, or buttocks. It often leads to a weakness in the legs. You usually need treatments for weakness or pain with medications, and some physical therapy. How your recovery is varies and hinges on the nerve damage present.

Diabetic Focal Neuropathy affects certain nerves and often appears suddenly. It can also appear in the head, torso, or your legs, and causes a great deal of muscle weakness,and/or pain. Signs of focal neuropathy include double vision, eye pain, severe pain in a certain area such as the back or legs, and Bell's Palsy which is weakness on one side of the face.

Overall, to prevent serious problems with neuropathies, it is wisest to control your blood sugars in as many ways as possible. Keeping them under that 140 mark is best, and really prevents this serious problem in the first place. **Autonomic Neuropathy** is a very complex nerve disorder and can frequently affect diabetics. Autonomic neuropathy type can affect each and every body system which I will cover here. The symptomatology varies widely. Depending on where this disease is attacking inside the body systems, are the areas where symptoms will clearly show up.

Symptomatology
Dizziness and fainting when standing may occur with hypotension, which is low blood pressure.

Sexual difficulty which can include ejaculation problems in men, or erectile dysfunction. Females may be having vaginal dryness and problems with orgasm.

Stomach emptying such as gastroparesis causes the stomach to have a lot of trouble letting go of food eaten, making it difficult to digest.

Problems with sweat glands which means trouble producing sweat, or else the opposite of producing too much sweat. The reason for this being that the body cannot regulate its temperature.

Eye problems with pupil reaction. This makes it hard for the eyes to adjust from light to dark and problems with driving at night.

Trouble with exercise. The heart rate doesn't change even in aerobic exercise, but stays the same way.

Hypoglycemic unawareness. This is a lack of feeling when the blood sugars are too low, and you do not realize you are low.
One of the main problems with this neuropathy is a **diabetic bladder**

A diabetic bladder means that the signal you need to empty your bladder fails from the nerves when you have no feelings there anymore. Diabetic neuropathy or bladder damages these nerves of the urinary sphincter. The stream of urine is weakened, and causes a person to be unable to urinate much. Infection of the bladder is therefore very common in this problem, and the only way to solve it is by self-catheterization of the bladder where the bladder can be completely emptied. Drinking a lot of fluids and going to the restroom every 2 hours also helps the problem. Drugs that help this problem are Urecholine or Duvoid. These pills increase the tone of muscle that helps the bladder to empty.

Diagnosing this problem
If it is suspected that you have this nerve disorder, the following tests may be ordered:

Breathing Tests This is to find out how well your heart rate responds to breathing exercises and how the blood pressure does as well.

Gastrointestinal Tests to determine how well your stomach empties or not. This usually means a GI series.

Tilt-Table Test which tells how well your body responds to different positions with blood pressure and heart rate.

QSART Test The QSART test stands for Quantitative sudomotor axon reflex test. It tells the story on how your nerves which are responsible for sweating will respond back when stimulated. They perform this test by a current that is electrical and small, and with capsule types that are placed on the extremities, you should feel a tingling. The **Thermoregulatory Test** might also be done which you are powdered with a special powder that changes color. The powder changes color when you sweat. They will place you in a special chamber, increasing temperature. Your temperature will go up at least 1 degree up to 1.5 degrees while there. Photographs are taken while in there to see your body's actual sweating. They can diagnose autonomic neuropathy easily by this test after seeing the sweating pattern, whether normal or abnormal.

A bladder ultrasound may be done to take bladder pictures.

Treating the whole picture of autonomic neuropathy involves what is causing the basic problem. Blood sugar control needs to be kept in tight control, and other drugs for the various problems throughout the body will need to be given.

For stomach trouble, the proper diet may help by adding some fiber-rich foods along with more fluids. Drugs that help stomach emptying also help the person to feel better, and lead a more productive life. One such drug is Reglan, which makes stomach emptying more productive.

For heart related problems in autonomic neuropathy, doctors may give a blood pressure pill that regulates your system. Other drugs that help your body keep the right amounts of salt may do a lot.

Medications to control sweating if you have that problem may be given. Drugs such as Clonidine for example, decrease the sweating problems.

Acupuncture is a Chinese healing practice that may actually ease the pain of neuropathy symptoms.

This has been a practice in China for at least 2,000 years or better. Needles that are very tiny and sterile, are placed into specific places on the body to ease pain and help wellness. This practice has grown in the US in the last many years now.

Acupuncture can have many benefits from helping people with nausea and vomiting after chemotherapy to post-surgical wellness.

People that have painful neuropathies from diabetes seem to benefit in many cases I have read. Diabetic peripheral neuropathy has been often been treated with several sessions of this Chinese practice, and people have shown a great improvement in their painful neuropathy symptoms. In fact, in a small percentage of persons, the symptomatology associated with neuropathy has totally cleared up.

It has been explored by health experts that this practice often works since many medical problems are caused by imbalances in the body systems. They say that there is a blockage causing these imbalances as there is in diabetic neuropathy, and that this practice helps the nervous systems making a natural flow in the meridians, which are nerves passages through the body. The nervous system becomes more regulated, and therefore, helping endorphins, which is the body's natural pain killing mechanism. Neurotransmitters are assisted as well since the brain chemistry is regulated by neurohormones.

If you think that this Chinese practice may help you, talk about it with your diabetes healthcare team.

PAD or Peripheral Arterial Disease as it stands for, is a type of neuropathy seen frequently in diabetics. It is said that type 2 diabetics are actually at a higher risk for developing PAD due to bodily changes that happen with diabetes. Insulin resistance puts the type 2 person at a higher risk. Arteries become clogged with fatty deposits. This leads to hardening of the arteries, and the blood vessels also narrow. The reason that this is more frequent in a type 2 diabetic is because in this type of diabetes, there is usually a higher level of fatty acids more than in type 1. But this is not to say it cannot happen in type 1 as well.

As mentioned before, types of neuropathies can cause decreased feelings in the legs and feet. This will in turn, cause a person not to notice small injuries to the foot such as a cut or blisters. When you continue to walk on the injury, it is highly possible that they will worsen and get bigger, becoming infected too. If you have a combination of both PAD and also other neuropathy, it multiplies more problems because your blood flowing to the feet gets reduced. This means that your body will have a difficult time healing or fighting any infections. Wounds that are not attended to, will then get a severe infection and even lead into an ulcer.

Even more can go wrong in PAD if your blood vessels which are in your heart or brain. This is what can rapidly, and without warning bring on strokes or heart attacks. Anyone living with peripheral arterial has about a 7 in 10 chance of having an amputation in the next 3-5 years.

The first symptom that you may have a problem with peripheral arterial disease is pain which comes in the legs, feet, or toes. It can wake you out of sound sleep, and increase when walking. If the pain lets up when you sit down, this is referred to as claudication. Other times the feeling is described as not pain, but a heaviness, tiredness, or else cramping that occurs in the thighs, buttocks, or calves. This discomfort and pain you are feeling can make you unable to carry out activities that you do daily such as shopping in the mall, or socializing.

Sometimes people experiencing peripheral arterial disease may notice that sores on the legs or feet have trouble with healing, or never heal at all.

When your feet are cold a lot, this can be another telltale sign.

Other signs of peripheral arterial disease may also include color changes in feet, poor nail growth, and decreased hair growth on your legs or toes.

There are times that it is a possibility that PAD has no symptoms. PAD in diabetics will often go after the smaller blood vessels below the knee. And at this place on the body, there is often nothing felt that is wrong.

How is this problem of peripheral arterial disease diagnosed?

Your doctor will ask you a series of questions to figure out your risk, and feel for pulses in the feet, and for other symptoms I mentioned of above. You would probably be given a test called an ankle-brachial index test. This test is painless and not invasive. It takes around 20-30 minutes, and you will need to lay down for about 10 minutes. The laying down for 10 minutes is so that the gravity effect is the same on your arms and legs. That way the results will come out accurately.

After the laying down, a doctor or nurse will measure your blood pressure numbers in your arms, and then in each foot a couple places. They'll measure it with a Doppler probe, which uses sound waves that can tell blood flow. The systolic number alone will be recorded for each area measured. They should compare the blood pressure readings in your ankles and then your arms. If it looks like it is lower in your ankles, then PAD is a strong possibility.

Since the ABI is just a screening test, it does not tell you anything about where a blockage may be located. So in order to find this information out, you would probably be referred to a vascular specialist for more tests. The medical tests done would probably be an MRI, and/or angiogram to look at the way your blood is flowing.

Once you find out you have peripheral arterial disease, there are some treatments available. A lot of times blood pressure drugs along with diabetes pills, and cholesterol lowering drugs will help this cause. You may also receive what is called an antiplatelet medication to cut the risk of clots developing in your blood vessels.

Surgery is another option for this medical issue. Angioplasty will open up arteries leading to the heart, but it can also be done to clear arteries leading to the heart. Artery bypass is another possibility to correct this situation, as another artery is taken from another place in the body, and is reattached around the section of a blocked artery.

Doctors can also do plaque removal. A small tube is inserted into whichever artery is affected . Then a tiny rotating blade will be used to take plaque from the wall of the artery. If the artery is really blocked up however, this is not usually an option.

Besides keeping your blood glucose under control, cholesterol lowering is very important to avoid this problem of peripheral artery disease. Smoking does not help either, as any smoker will have a very high chance of developing this serious complication.

Article contributed by Elinor Nauen on PAD

You walk a block, then clutch your leg with what feels like a charley horse. You stop, and the pain does too. The discomfort may be a warning of a common yet serious condition called peripheral arterial disease (PAD).

In PAD, the same fatty material that can clog heart arteries builds up in the arteries of the legs, blocking blood flow. The risk for death from heart attack or stroke is six to seven times greater in people with PAD—equivalent to the risk of someone who's had a heart attack or stroke. Without prompt treatment, one in four people with the condition will suffer a heart attack, stroke or amputation or die within five years.

PAD is most often recognized when it causes claudication—fatigue, cramps, tiredness or pain in the leg or buttock muscles that goes away when you stop walking. Less frequently, PAD can cause ulcers or slow-healing wounds on the feet or toes, or pain in the feet or toes that disturbs sleep. However, as many as half to two thirds of those with the condition have no symptoms.

As with coronary heart disease, key risk factors for PAD are having diabetes, smoking or having smoked, and being over age 50. "If you have no other risk factors, age alone will increase risk—and yet risk rapidly increases even in younger people who smoke or have diabetes," says Alan T. Hirsch, M.D., professor of epidemiology at the University of Minnesota School of Public Health in Minneapolis. "We want people to recognize that if you are over 50 and have any other risk factor, you have a one in four chance of having PAD."

Also at risk are African Americans and anyone with chronic kidney disease, high blood pressure, high blood cholesterol or a personal or family history of vascular disease, heart attack or stroke. An estimated 8 to 12 million people in this country have PAD.

If you have risk factors, talk to your doctor, whether or not you have symptoms. The PAD Coalition, a consortium of health organizations and government agencies, recommends that those at risk get a quick, painless, accurate and inexpensive diagnostic test called an ABI (ankle-brachial index).

The good news: PAD is both preventable and treatable. "PAD is a common and serious disease, which merits immediate and lifelong attention," says Dr. Hirsch. "Become informed and take actions to protect your health."

ARMS FOR LEGS

While exercise is helpful for people with PAD, walking—a typical workout for sufferers—can also be painful. Diane Treat-Jacobson, R.N., Ph.D., assistant professor at the University of Minnesota in Minneapolis, has done studies on the effects of exercise on people with PAD. She recently discovered that supervised training using aerobic arm exercise was as beneficial as treadmill walking in improving walking distance. Treat-Jacobson notes that while results are preliminary, arm exercise might be a pain-free option that can "help break the cycle of disability or enable patients to start exercising sooner after a surgical procedure."

Another Article by a retired podiatrist Dr. Michael, MD I thought would be

valuable:

I am a retired Podiatrist, who for 15 years worked predominantly with patients diagnosed with diabetes. The risk factors affecting the lower extremities among diabetic patients include a potential for the loss of protective sensation, and an acceleration of atherosclerosis (clogging of the arteries) leading to an early onset of peripheral vascular disease. Both of these clinical entities increase the risk of wound development and loss of limb. The loss of sensation, known as peripheral neuropathy essentially raises the individual's pain threshold so that they will either have a delayed reaction to an injury, or at the extreme, feel no pain whatsoever. Let's examine the responses of an individual with impaired sensation versus another with normal sensation, both wearing shoes with a defect in the innersole producing excessive friction. Our normal subject would experience pain within 2 minutes of putting the shoes on, and would remove them to find an area which was slightly irritated, but the skin unbroken. Our neuropathic walker could conceivably complete his half hour walk before noting some mild discomfort. Upon removing his shoes he might find blistering, or a frank break in the integrity of the skin. Your physician can determine if your protective sensation has been impacted through the use of a simple kit, known as the Semmes Weinstein monofilament test. This kit was originally developed to test the level of protective sensation in patients suffering with Hansen's disease (aka leprosy) who are also subject to neuropathy. The kit consists of flexible plastic monofilaments of differing diameter, the ability to perceive the touch of the smaller diameter fibers (with eyes closed) measures an individual's ability to respond to painful stimuli. Fortunately, with tight control of blood sugars it is possible to avoid or delay the onset of diabetic neuropathy.

Chronic Kidney Disease

Chronic kidney disease is an all too common factor in diabetics. High blood glucose destroys the filters in each kidney over time, and thus begins the loss of function. Chronic kidney disease has stages which I am going to describe in this article and what happens as the kidneys slowly decline. There will also be video discussions of kidney disease and the dialysis process.

What are the stages of chronic kidney disease?
Stage 1-In stage 1, there is very mild kidney damage with normal or high GFR (glomerular filtration rate) of 90 ML or more. There is really not much to panic about at this point as kidneys are doing pretty good.

Stage 2-With stage 2, there will be a mild decrease in GFR, and some mild kidney damage has taken place at this point. The GFR score is usually between 60-89, still not too bad, but needs to be rechecked every so often with a blood creatinine test.

Stage 3-In stage 3, things are getting a little more serious. There is another decrease in the GFR rate, which is between 30-59 ML. You may start seeing blood test results show anemia, which is a shortage of red blood cells, and early bone disease may peak. This is where some treatment should begin to reduce more bone troubles and iron given for the anemia present.

Stage 4-Stage 4 is very serious. It now means time to think about dialysis. You may feel unwell, have itchy skin, many kidney infections, or urinary tract problems by now. There may also be blood in the urine, and less urine produced.

Stage 5-Kidney failure is beginning in stage 5 and chances are you will not feel well, have itchy skin all the time, not be urinating much, if at all, (maybe a teaspoon per day), have nausea, headaches, and vomiting. Pushing a lot of fluids will make this problem worse at this point when urination has come to almost a complete stop. It is now referred to as ESRD which stands for end stage renal disease.

So as you can see, kidney disease does **NOT** have too many symptoms until the later stages of progression. You can slow this progression down by controlling your blood sugars, and watching your hemoglobin A1C levels every three months.

To elaborate more on creatinine. Creatinine is a waste that healthy kidneys are able to remove from your blood. A creatinine clearance test is done by taking a 24-hour urine sample and a blood sample. This test will calculate how quickly your kidneys clear your blood of this waste product. The other way to measure creatinine clearance is to have a blood creatinine test which measures the GFR as I mentioned above. The GFR rate tells how quickly, or slowly, your kidneys are cleaning your blood. If your kidneys are entirely normal functioning, then your GFR should not really be under 90 or better.

If your kidney's are declining at stage 3 or more, you really need to be under the care of a nephrologist, which is a kidney specialist. A kidney doctor like this can help you slow the rate of decline of your kidney function, decide if you may or may not need a kidney biopsy, diagnose for sure the type of kidney trouble you are having, and manage complications of CKD such as anemia, hypertension, metabolic acidosis, and your body's vitamin and mineral balance. Dialysis can hopefully be delayed for a long time, and also with the proper diet with CKD. Hemoglobin A1C helps detect diabetic problems.

The Kidney Diet

The kidney diet is a bit restrictive in many areas, but you can still find food and recipes that are satisfying to eat.

This special kidney diet helps you to manage your blood sugar levels, and also help reduce the amount of unwanted waste your kidneys process, along with fluids. You and your dietitian will work out the exchanges of protein, fat, and carbohydrates that you will need on a daily basis. Your sodium, phosphorus, and potassium will also have to be worked out in your meal plan since you don't process these nutritional elements correctly any longer.

Portion control in this diet plan is essential. You will need to accurately weigh many foods to get the right serving size.

Your food labels are important sources of information on your renal diet. Many choices such as diet colas, peanut butter, some cereals, and even lemonades and teas are loaded with sodium and phosphorus.
Eating your meals on your renal diet plan at the same time each day is important, just as it is for your diabetes anyway. Spacing out your food allowances is important to allow you more flexibility in snacking.
Below is a list of foods that are recommended:

Milk that is skim or fat-free; Non-dairy creamer, plain yogurts, sugar-free puddings, sugar free ice-creams, and sugar-free non-dairy desserts.

White bread, unsweetened refined dry cereals, cream of wheat, grits, noodles, pastas, rices, bagel (small), hamburger bun, unsalted crackers, cornbread made from scratch, flour tortillas.

Apples are allowed along with apple juice, applesauce, apricot halves, strawberries, blackberries and blueberries. You can also have low-sugar cranberry juice, cherries and fruit cocktail, grapefruit, grapes, grape juice, kumquats, oranges, pears, pineapples, plums, tangerines and watermelons.

For starchy vegetables eating corn, peas, mixed vegetables with corn and peas in moderation, as they are high in phosphorus. You can have potatoes that are soaked to reduce potassium. See video on this.
For non-starchy vegetables, you can have asparagus beets, broccoli, brussel sprouts, carrots,celery, cabbage, cauliflower, eggplant, frozen broccoli, green beans iceberg lettuce, kale, leeks, mustard greens, onions, okra, red and green peppers, raw spinach, radishes, snow peas, summer

squash and turnips.

Foods you should avoid are these listed. If consumed, they will worsen your renal problems. They are:

Chocolate milk, buttermilk, sweetened yogurt, sugar-sweetened pudding, ice cream with sugar, sugared nondairy frozen desserts.
On the breads list of forbidden foods are whole wheat bread, sugary cereals, bran, granola or whole wheat cereals, instant cereals, whole grain hot cereals,gingerbread, pancake mix, cornbread mix, biscuits, salty snacks like potato chips, corn chips, peanuts and crackers.

On fruits you must avoid avocados, bananas, cantaloupes, dried fruits such as raisins, dates, prunes and fresh pears. Honeydew melons, kiwis, star fruit, kumquats, mangoes, papaya, nectarines, oranges, and orange juice and pomegranate are all things to stay away from.

Baked potatoes, sweet potatoes, yams, baked beans, dried beans, succotash, pumpkin and winter squash are starches to be avoided.

Artichokes, fresh bamboo shoots, beet greens, cactus, cooked Chinese cabbages, rutabagas, sauerkraut, cooked spinach, tomatoes, tomato sauce or paste, tomato juice, and vegetable juices must all be avoided.

On the higher protein foods, you can eat things like lean cuts of meat, poultry, fish and seafood, eggs or egg substitutes. You can eat limited amounts of cottage cheese due to high sodium.

You must avoid bacon, canned and luncheon meats, cheeses, hot dogs, liver, nuts, pepperoni, salami, salmon and sausages. These all have sodium counts that are too high.

For higher fat foods in your condiments it is best to choose soft or tub margarine that is low in trans fats. You can also choose low-fat mayonnaise, low-fat sour cream, and low fat cream cheese. It is best to avoid bacon fat, butter, Crisco, shortening, whipping cream, and margarines which are high in trans fats.

For your beverage selections which will be limited daily according to how much fluid you still put out, it is best to have clear diet sodas, homemade tea, water, or Crystal Light. You should avoid having dark colas like Coke, Pepsi, or Root Beer. Fruit juices are not good either of any type. Many of these juices have phosphoric acids which the kidneys rebel against when they are failing.

Other foods to strictly limit or not have at all are candies, syrups, honey, molasses, pies, cakes, cookies, and donuts. Your sauces like barbecue, and ketchup must be avoided. TV dinners are bad choices since they do contain a lot of sodium.

Urinary tract and kidney problems are extremely common in both cases of type 1 and type 2 diabetes. Diabetic nephropathy is a common complication. This means that your kidney loses its ability to function the way it should. The first laboratory sign on a urinalysis is proteinuria, (protein in the urine). Another medical term for this condition is also known as Kimmelstiel-Wilson disease, or diabetic glomerulosclerosis. As I had mentioned in a previous article link to this one, each of your kidneys is made up of hundreds of thousands of nephrons. The nephrons are a cluster of blood vessels called a glomerulus. The glomeruli is supposed to filter blood and then form your urine. The urine in turn, should drain down into the ureter.

When the glomerulus thickens, the kidney may begin to dysfunction by allowing more albumin which is protein to slip out. There is a simple test to detect this problem called a microalbuminuria test. If the level is over 30 after a 24 hour urine collection, this indicates a problem within the kidneys.

When diabetic nephropathy goes on progressing, the glomeruli are destroyed in increasing numbers. Thus, the levels of albumin increases. Protein released into the urine may show up many years before you actually have other symptoms. Hypertension will often go with nephropathy. As more time passes, the kidney's abilities to work properly start declining, sometimes rapidly. Diabetic nephropathy can then get into chronic kidney failure until you have reached ESRD, which is End Stage Renal Disease. This happens usually within a 2-5 year time period after proteinuria.

Early stage diabetic nephropathy is known to be silent, and has no symptoms. Signs of this complication often don't appear until you have reached more acute renal failure. What you will probably notice then besides not feeling well, are:

fatigue-being too tired
foamy, or frothy urine
hiccups all the time
itchy skin all the time
nausea and vomiting in the acute stage
swelling of the legs and puffiness in the face
lack of any appetite
Hypertension may be present

The goal once nephropathy is discovered is to slow it down along with other related complications. Once proteinuria is found, the blood pressure must also be kept in control by medications. Medicines such as angiotensin converting enzymes or angiotensin receptor blockers, are the medications of choice. These types of medications will reduce the diabetic nephropathy.

Over the counter drugs used to treat pain such as Ibuprofen, and Naproxen may injure the weakened kidneys. For alternatives on pain drugs, always ask your physician.

Urinary tract or bladder dysfunction can also be a contributing factor to kidney diseases. Diabetes can damage nerves that control the bladder muscles. Both men and women with diabetes often have urinary urgency, frequency, or leakage of urine.

More severe symptoms include having a difficult time urinating and incomplete bladder emptying. These signs are indicative of what is known as neurogenic bladder. Your doctor should check out your nervous system, (this means the brain and the bladder nerves themselves). And your doctor may also run tests that include an IVP, (kidney test with dye), other xrays, and a general urological evaluation called urodynamics.

Treating a neurogenic bladder usually involves self catheterization when the biggest problem present is fluid retention in the bladder. And if urine leakage becomes too big a problem, then surgical procedures may help.

Urinary tract infections are also another problem for the diabetic. They occur when too much bacteria usually enter the urinary tract. If bacteria are growing in the urethra, the infection is known as urethritis. The bacteria will sometimes go on up into the body and cause something more serious called pyelonephritis, a kidney infection. Signs of a urinary tract infection might be:

a frequent urge to urinate
pain or burning in the bladder/urethra during urination
bloody urine, (hematuria)
pressure above the pubic bone in women
feeling of fullness in the rectum for men
When the infection is present in the kidneys, you may be nauseated, and feel flank pain in your back. A fever will usually accompany kidney infections.

Treating the infection as soon as possible is vitally important. When these problems become too big, they can cause a shutdown of the whole urinary system, and kidneys may quit functioning as well.

The Dialysis Process and How it Works

venous catheter, two tubes will be connected to the blood transport tubes that are The biggest job of the kidneys is to filter wastes and produce urine. But when kidneys slack off, and begin to fail, they will no longer make anymore urine or get rid of toxins inside the body. Toxins build up and then there is a condition called uremia, a fancy name for renal failure. Hemodialysis is one way of replacing your kidney function until a transplant becomes available that is a suitable match.

With the process of hemodialysis, your blood is removed from your body, cleaned with dialysate, (the artificial kidney fluid), and returned to you. On the average, a person has around 10-12 pints of blood. During the hemodialysis procedure, only a little bit of blood, (1 pint at a time), is removed from your body to the dialyzer, cleaned by the artificial kidney dialysate and returned to you.

For access to get dialysis treatments, you will need a port of some type. They are arteriovenous fistula, or arteriovenous graft, or a central venous catheter. The most recommended is usually the AV fistula. You and your nephrologist will decide what's best though.

The first thing that happens in hemodialysis is the nurse or technician will take your blood pressure and other vitals. Your weight is also recorded, which tells how much excess fluid you need to have removed during the dialyzing process. You then go to the dialyzer and get hooked up to the machine. If you have a central venous catheter attached to the dialyzer and back into the body from there after processing. The dialyzer is programmed to your needs.

The dialysis machine keeps track of your blood flow, blood pressure, (some people get really low blood pressure), and how much fluid is being taken from your body. The blood does not go through the dialysis machine. The dialysis machine mixes dialysate solution, the fluid that goes into it. This fluid pulls out toxins from the blood, and then the bath goes down the drain. A blood pump is in the machine that keeps the blood flowing by creating a pumping action on the blood tubes that carry the uncleansed blood from the body, and then back to you after the "bath."

Hemodialysis is usually done three times a week for 4-5 hours each time.

Proteinuria Explained

Proteinuria is a sign of protein in the urine which signifies early kidney disease. One of the most frequent complications in both diabetic types is nephropathy. Nephropathy develops slowly over many years time. Eventually, **the kidney function fails, and dialysis is needed**. Your kidneys, as previously mentioned in other site articles here, filter wastes and toxins from the body.

Clinical albuminuria will often get into serious kidney disease after a number of years go by, anywhere from 5 or more. Good preventive practice is to monitor with laboratory urine tests for microalbuminuria and catch early filter problems. If this problem is seen at the early stages, there are things to be done to prevent worsening of the problems.

Tight control of blood sugar is very important. This cuts the risk of the kidneys having to take further abuse from high blood sugars.
Hypertension control , is also very important early on since hypertension injures nephrons the higher the blood pressure goes, and therefore causes proteinuria.

Blood pressure pills that have an angiotensin converting enzyme can stop kidney disease progression by slowing the leaking of protein in the urine.

Lower protein diets may or may not be helpful. There is research that suggests it has been helpful.

Treating **urinary tract infections** is a must. This problem is often a problem for many diabetic people. When a urinary tract infection is left untreated, it can definitely cause kidney scarring, and kill the nephron's functions further still. Over time with multiple bladder or urinary tract problems, this causes great kidney injury, and therefore the filtering ability becomes very damaged or not working at all. Taking cranberry pills cuts down on the urinary tract infection factor for many people. The acid factor in these pills you can get over the counter kills certain types of bladder infections.

Contribution by Jason Colling

Bladder infection is the word, which can strike fear in the eyes of everyone just by listening it. It can be said for a person who had this problem before or who has seen others in the past. It is one of the most painful infections. In this problem a person has to go to the urinal frequently and some time the urinal might be a painful one, which is enough to make anyone off.

Therefore it should be fully treated as early as possible. But before that it should be diagnosed early. If this infection is diagnosed early than the person can be treated very fast and this infection can be easily disposed off by taking some medicine and you can make it a past thing. It is important to identifying and treating bladder infection, so that you could eliminate it from the urinary tract.

Urinary tract is the most important part of your body; it is the one which interacts with urine and tangentially, the kidney and liver. It is also a place where the bladder infection occurs. So when the urinary tract system fails then there is no other way from where you can interact with the kidney and liver and here the problems started to come. One of the main cause for bladder infections are the blockages in the bladder, which helps to maintain the urine flow and prevents the bladder from emptying completely. The remaining urine in the bladder increases the chance of multiplying the bacteria can cause an infection in the bladder. These bacteria's are bad, they are the main culprit who blocks the bladder and gives problem to a person. In most case of bladder infection two main bad bacteria's are e-coli or human feces.

There are some preventions can be done, so that you will not have these problems in the future. Like you should drink lots of water in a day, so that your system should remain clean, do not wear tight clothes, avoid taking the caffeine beverages etc. If you keep all these in mind then there is very chance remained of any bladder infection.

There are some infection which can come at any time in your body and one the most painful infection is Bladder infection. In this infection a person bladder gets blocked by the bad bacteria like e-coli or human feces and they can cause many problems in your urinal system. Therefore it should be treated as soon as possible. One of the fortunate parts is that this infection can be fully treated in a very less period depending upon the stage of the infection. You can also take some preventions so that you won't get this infection in future.

Article contribution by Krishan B Kinar

Guidelines for the Prevention of Urinary Tract Infection (UTI)
From the foregoing information on UTI, one should realize that the best course is to follow, strictly, the preventive measures, which are very simple, mostly relating to routine hygiene, rather than being on long-term prophylactic antibiotics; or, in neglected cases, developing terminal kidney disease, i.e. kidney failure, which may, require repeated dialysis, or even kidney transplant, depending on the case.

Various guidelines are mentioned below, and all individuals, irrespective of age and sex, are required to carefully follow them in their everyday life.

(i) Perineal hygiene

The perineum is the area where the openings of the anus, the urethra and the vagina are situated (of course, the scrotum and the penis in the male). It is the most dangerous area, especially in females, as all the three openings are lying close together (Fig. 21), and there is always a threat of infection to the urinary tract from anal-faecal organisms, which invade the urinary tract through the urethral opening. Hence if proper hygiene is maintained after each defecation, the infection from the anus to the urethra can be stopped/prevented since UTI is caused mostly by E. coli organisms present in the faeces. Of course, the various predisposing/associated factors responsible for UTI, if present, have to be simultaneously investigated and treated.

A simple cleansing with water, and preferably with soap and water after passing stools, and urine in the case of females, is strongly recommended at all ages, more so in children, girls, both married and unmarried women. However, those using toilet-paper, after passing stools, should be more careful, and see that the area has been thoroughly cleaned, especially in the case of females. Hence, it is of the utmost importance to always keep the perineal area clean, and thus it has been rightly said that 'cleanliness is next to godliness.'

(ii) Passing of urine after sexual intercourse (postcoital voiding) Since during sexual activity, the organisms may gain entry through the urethral opening into the urinary bladder, it is advisable for all women to pass urine after each sexual intercourse, so that the bacteria, in case they have entered the urinary bladder, are washed out. It is safer if urine is also passed before sexual intercourse.

Further, women who are more prone to UTI, or get recurrences of UTI as a result of intercourse, are advised to take a single dose of prophylactic broad-spectrum antibiotic like norfloxacin, ciprofloxacin, lomefloxacin or ofloxacin, etc., after sexual intercourse/ coitus. This is an important step in the prevention of UTI in such patients, and has shown promising results. .

The above step for the prevention of UTI is very important and calls for an urgent need to impart sex education at the appropriate age. Physicians / obstetricians / gynaecologists / paediatricians can also guide their patients as and when an opportunity arises. Mothers can also advise their children in this matter.

(iii) Passing of urine frequently

All persons, and especially those who are more prone to UTI, should pass urine frequently, say every 3-4 hours, so that the urinary bladder is constantly washed out, and the bacteria, if any, are pushed out in the urine. If the bladder is not evacuated frequently, the bacteria will get more time to increase in number in the urine collected in the urinary bladder. Hence, frequent urination is an essential step towards the prevention of UTI, which should be observed by everyone.

In any case, urination should not be postponed, as this will increase the rise of UTI.

(iv) Passing of urine at bedtime

Similarly, urine must be passed at bedtime, so that the minimum quantity of urine remains in the urinary bladder during the night. Since the duration of the night is long, there should be as little urine as possible in the bladder, and one should pass urine even during the night, if he or she happens to wake up.

(v) Plenty of fluids

It is obvious that the intake of plenty of fluids is required, so that there is frequent urination, and the bladder is constantly kept clean. At least about three litres of water/fluids must be taken daily to achieve the desired results.

Ideally, the habit of frequent urination or bladder training, including cleanliness, should be instilled right from childhood, especially in the case of female children. Above all, once the subject is made clear to the sufferers/others, it becomes routine.

(vi) Immediate treatment of predisposing factors

As soon as some predisposing/ obstructive lesions happen to occur, e.g. urinary stones, benign enlargement of prostate, etc., immediate attention should be paid, and surgery, if required, should not be delayed, so that UTI does not develop at all, and there is absolute prevention.

(vii) Control of high blood pressure and diabetes

Control of high blood pressure and diabetes is an essential requirement to prevent the kidneys from contracting an infection, since a damaged kidney, as a result of high blood pressure and/or high blood sugar, is always prone to get infection. The infection in such kidneys can only be avoided/ prevented if it is protected from damage by these diseases. That is, a strict control of both high blood pressure and diabetes is required. This aspect has also been emphasized earlier.

Skin Problems Related to Diabetes

Skin disorders can affect people with both types of diabetes. Many people with both type 1 and 2 diabetes will have some type of skin disorder that is brought on by diabetes. Sometimes this is a signal you may have diabetes and not know it. Many of your skin conditions can be easily prevented or easily corrected if caught early.

Bacterial infection, fungal-type infections, or itching are of the most common types. Some of the most common are called styes. Styes are infections of the glands in the eyelid. Boils, or infections in the hair follicles are skin types of infection. The other type of deep infection deep inside the skin is carbuncles.

Tissues that are inflamed will usually be hot to the touch. There is also swelling and redness present, along with pain. Different organisms can cause infections. The most common ones are Staphylococcus bacteria that is also called a staph infection.

At one point in our history, these bacterial infections of the skin were of a life-threatening nature. But today of course, antibiotics of all types are available to cure all types of serious skin complications.

Now fungal infections in those with diabetes are often referred to as **Candida albicans**. This is a yeast like fungus that creates itchy rashes in moist red areas that are usually surrounded by blisters and scales. These infections thrive in warm moist folds of the skin. These problematic parts of the body are usually around the nails, the breasts, and between fingers and toes. It can also come up in corners of the mouth, the groin, and armpits. The more common fungal infections are athlete's foot, ringworm, vaginal infections, and jock itch.

Skin disorders of itching are often brought on by diabetes. They are usually in the form of a yeast infection, dry skin, or poor circulation. If poor circulation is the cause of itching, the itchiest areas may be the legs. You can usually treat itching yourself. Limit how often you bathe.

Use mild soap with a moisturizer and apply skin creams after bathing that are gentle.

Diabetic Dermopathy is a skin disorder that causes changes in the small blood vessels. Dermopathy will usually look like light brown scaly patches. Many people think that these are age spots. This skin problem reflects itself in the front of your legs. The patches really are not painful, or will open up. There is also no itching. Dermopathy is not an emergency.

Atherosclerosis is a thickening of the arteries. It likes to get into the legs. People with diabetes tend to get this condition at younger ages. Atherosclerosis is very serious because it will narrow the blood vessels. The skin will change, become hairless, thin, cool, and also shiny. Your toes will be cold, and toenails discolor and thicken. Exercising causes pain in the calf muscles. The reason for this is that the muscles do not get enough oxygen.

Allergic skin reactions can occur sometimes from response to medications or insulins. If you think you are having some type of allergic skin reaction, it is best to talk to your doctor, and get treatment.

Treating your skin is another important part of your diabetes care and treatment. It is always best to practice preventive care before these types of complications set in. Talk to your doctor about what is best for your own skin care.

Tissues that are inflamed will usually be hot to the touch. There is also swelling and redness present, along with pain. Different organisms can cause infections. The most common ones are Staphylococcus bacteria that is also called a staph infection.

At one point in our history, these bacterial infections of the skin were of a life-threatening nature. But today of course, antibiotics of all types are available to cure all types of serious skin complications.

Now fungal infections in those with diabetes are often referred to as Candida albicans. This is a yeast like fungus that creates itchy rashes in moist red areas that are usually surrounded by blisters and scales. These infections thrive in warm moist folds of the skin. These problematic parts of the body are usually around the nails, the breasts, and between fingers and toes. It can also come up in corners of the mouth, the groin, and armpits. The more common fungal infections are athlete's foot, ringworm, vaginal infections, and jock itch.

Skin disorders of itching are often brought on by diabetes. They are usually in the form of a yeast infection, dry skin, or poor circulation. If poor circulation is the cause of itching, the itchiest areas may be the legs. You can usually treat itching yourself. Limit how often you bathe. Use mild soap with a moisturizer and apply skin creams after bathing that are gentle.

Necrobiosis Lipoidica

Necrobiosis is a skin disorder mostly seen in a diabetic. This skin disorder shows itself with red-brown papules and will usually turn into yellowish-brown plaques with central atrophy. It is usually on the lower extremities. It is not as common for this skin problem to occur in the upper extremities, meaning the face and scalp.

Necrobiosis lipoidica is a type of chronic dermatitis that is associated with Type 1 diabetes. It can happen in type 2 cases, but more rarely. Unless the lesions are really ulcerated, they are not symptomatic. This skin disorder usually happens between ages 30-40, but that doesn't mean it cannot happen at any age. It seems to appear more frequently in females than in males. It seems that there is really no relation to a person's blood sugar control and the chances of developing this problem. But I've read that diabetic people have much higher chances of getting this problem.

Collagen and this ulcerative skin problem has seemed to show a connection to this problem. Diabetics have collagen problems in some complications such as trigger finger and frozen shoulder problems. As of yet, there is no treatment that can really clear up this problem, but topical glucocorticoids for the earlier lesions on the skin have been shown to help. Systemic cyclosporine has been another favorable treatment as well as using aspirin therapies.

Heart Health and Diabetes

Heart disease is common in people with diabetes.
A diabetic is at least two to four times more likely to have coronary artery disease. And once a person with diabetes has a heart or stroke event, it is very likely that it will recur again. Many diabetics are unaware of this statistic.

Since diabetics are at higher risk for heart disease and stroke, which are leading causes of death in the United States and Canada, prevention of all three of these dangerous conditions is very important.

When you have diabetes, it is important to do whatever you can to maintain a healthy heart. Diabetes causes heart disease because of the chemical changes in the blood. And then these changes make it very simple for fatty acids, (known as plaque), to form on the blood vessel walls. When this happens, you then have what is called premature atherosclerosis, or more simply called hardening of the arteries. This hardening of the arteries is how the blood vessels become narrow. They can also clog up completely, causing a massive heart attack.

If you smoke, you really should quit as this makes your risk for heart-related events that much higher. Obesity and lack of physical activity, and insulin resistance are other contributing risk factors for heart trouble.

Good target cholesterol levels for diabetics
Women should have an HDL of 40 mg/dl and an LDL of <100 mg dl
Men should have an HDL of 50 mg/dl and an LDL of <100 mg/dl
Healthy Heart Tips to Follow

Exercise by walking even for only 15 minutes per day each day. Activity is good and increases your heart rate, which keeps you heart-healthy. Walking even decreases blood sugar levels.

Have regular cholesterol, lipid, and triglyceride testing. Not only is your blood sugar important, but lipids, cholesterol, and triglycerides are critical if you have diabetes, and even if you don't actually. Those blood components can and **DO** cause massive heart attacks or even a fast death if not treated properly.

Always remember your diet as well when you are diabetic. Diet is a big factor in helping cholesterol, lipids, and triglycerides stay where they are supposed to. If you keep them in check, you should live a longer, and healthier life.

This article was written by Scott Myers that I wanted to share on diabetes and circulatory disease.

Diabetes is a scourge on our society. The number of diabetes patients in the US has climbed to an estimated 12-14 million, up from 8 million in 1990. This article will deal with the growth in Type-I and Type-II diabetes in the US, and the effect that diabetes can have on circulatory disease.

The rate of increase is closely tied to the number of obese and morbidly obese people in the US. There are 66 million obese people in the US (obesity is defined as a BMI of over 30%). Nearly a fifth of these people have diabetes today. Left untreated, we can forecast that many with long-term obesity problems will eventually contract Type-II diabetes as a response to long-term problems of insulin resistance.

It's no coincidence, therefore, that rates of heart disease and other circulatory problems is increasing. What is surprising is, until recently, the rate of heart disease had been declining since the 1950's. The reason for the fall was primarily due to a reduction in cigarette smoking, from over 60% of the population, to under 25% today.

In addition, we've seen an increase in certain populations which are more susceptible to circulatory disease: these maladies are much more common amongst people of Latin American and African-American subgroups. There is a certain correlation between diabetes and circulatory disease. Both African-Americans and Latinos have much higher rates of obesity and heart disease. As those subgroups have grown, so has the overall incidence of diabetes and circulatory disease.

Finally, people are living longer. As we age, we grow more susceptible to circulatory diseases. It is estimated that the number of people in the US over 75 will double between 2005 and 2030.

What is the connection between diabetes and circulatory disease? Cause and effect works in two directions: as we exercise less, we gain weight. With less exercise, we also tend to have higher levels of circulating insulin. These higher levels contribute to an overall increase in insulin resistance from the cells of the body. As insulin resistance increases, the pancreas increases insulin output in order to counteract the problem. A long period of insulin resistance is typically followed by the onset of insulin-resistant Type-II diabetes.

What effect does diabetes have on the circulatory system? Blood vessels thicken throughout the body in response two three factors related to obesity and diabetes:

High blood pressure causes a thickening of the arteries

High circulating LDL and lower HDL ratios contribute to the formation of plaque in blood vessels, which leads to a further narrowing of those vessels

Inflammation, which can result from circulating substances such as homocysteine in obese and diabetic patients, leads to higher levels of heart and circulatory disease.

The smaller the blood vessels, the greater the damage caused by this thickening and narrowing of the blood vessels. The greatest problem in both diabetics and obese people is with their circulation in the capillaries and their extremities. That's why we see blindness (as a result of constriction in the capillaries of the eye), neuropathy in the feet and hands, and a reduction in circulation in the brain and heart, all are due to a less-effective circulation and narrowing of the arteries.

Heart disease and circulatory disease are interrelated. It is estimated that 60% of those patients who undergo angioplasty will also need vascular intervention, particularly in the kidneys, iliac, SFA (superficial femoral artery) and femoral-popliteal arteries of the leg. Left untreated, patients are at a much higher risk of heart attacks, strokes, and diabetic foot ulcers.

Diabetes is closely linked to heart and other circulatory diseases. The correlation between the two means that both must be treated in order to improve a person's morbidity and mortality.

Diabetic cardiomyopathy is a result of damage to the heart functions. Diabetics of both types have an extremely high rate of this problem occurring. In fact, I've read that around 52% of people with type 2 have this heart problem.

How does diabetes affect the heart muscle to cause cardiomyopathy? First of all, the heart has four chambers. There are two chambers on top, and another two on the bottom. These are called your heart ventricles. Every time the heart beats, these chambers will contract in a synchronized fashion. The atria will contract, filling the ventricles with blood. The next step is that the ventricles of the heart contract, which sends blood circulating. Then the cycle happens repeatedly, as each time the atria relax and fills with blood again.

Doctors over the years have done much study, noticing the changes in the structure and heart functions, especially in diabetic people. Left ventricle diastolic dysfunction is one of the main symptoms of this diabetic heart trouble. This is impairment in the way the left ventricle will fill with blood in between heartbeats, along with the increased filling on the part of the atria. This is an abnormality, and the heart will often become enlarged. This is diagnosed by doctors as left ventricular hypertrophy. This heart problem is brought on largely by insulin is a result of damage to the heart functions. Diabetics of both types have an extremely high rate of this problem occurring. In fact, I've read that around 52% of people with type 2 have this heart problem.

How does diabetes affect the heart muscle to cause cardiomyopathy? First of all, the heart has four chambers. There are two chambers on top, and another two on the bottom. These are called your heart ventricles. Every time the heart beats, these chambers will contract in a synchronized fashion. The atria will contract, filling the ventricles with blood. The next step is that the ventricles of the heart contract, which sends blood circulating. Then the cycle happens repeatedly, as each time the atria relax and fills with blood again.

Doctors over the years have done much study, noticing the changes in the structure and heart functions, especially in diabetic people. Left ventricle diastolic dysfunction is one of the main symptoms of this diabetic heart trouble. This is impairment in the way the left ventricle will fill with blood in between heartbeats, along with the increased filling on the part of the atria. This is an abnormality, and the heart will often become enlarged. This is diagnosed by doctors as left ventricular hypertrophy. This heart problem is brought on largely by insulin resistance syndrome.

Myocardial fibrosis is another problem that is often seen in diabetics. This is a scarring that occurs in the thick middle layer of your heart wall, which is the myocardium. Myocardial fibrosis is often due to the high blood glucose levels, which sets off damages and glycation of proteins in the myocardium.

This is why measurement of hemoglobin A1C is important to know every 3 months for diabetics. It helps to keep aware of these possible heart complications. Since type 2 diabetics as well as type 1 are known to have problems with diabetic cardiomyopathy, doctors and researchers in the medical field are calling for more awareness in screening for this problem. The best screening methods are not agreed on that I have read about yet. But there has been some connection with microalbuminuria, which is protein in the urine, to be connected somehow with diabetic diastolic dysfunction. Ask your doctor about this theory.

Echocardiography gives more of a clear picture of what condition your heart is in, and tells your cardiologist and doctor exactly more of what is taking place inside there.

There are a number of medications that doctors can use to head off cardiomyopathy from going into massive heart attacks and heart failure.

This is also again why good blood sugar control is very very important to your better health, and decreasing insulin resistance. The drugs called ACE inhibitors, which means angiotensin converting enzymes, lower your blood pressure. They are also used to decrease your chances of having myocardial fibrosis as well.

Beta blockers even in small doses help the heart up to a large degree sometimes, and decrease your chances of cardiomyopathy in the future. researchers in the medical field are calling for more awareness in screening for this problem. The best screening methods are not agreed on that I have read about yet. But there has been some connection with microalbuminuria, which is protein in the urine, to be connected somehow with diabetic diastolic dysfunction. Ask your doctor about this theory.

Echocardiography gives more of a clear picture of what condition your heart is in, and tells your cardiologist and doctor exactly more of what is taking place inside there.

There are a number of medications that doctors can use to head off cardiomyopathy from going into massive heart attacks and heart failure. This is also again why good blood sugar control is very very important to your better health, and decreasing insulin resistance. The drugs called ACE inhibitors, which means angiotensin converting enzymes, lower your blood pressure. They are also used to decrease your chances of having myocardial fibrosis as well. Beta blockers even in small doses help the heart up to a large degree sometimes, and decrease your chances of cardiomyopathy in the future.

Myocardial fibrosis is another problem that is often seen in diabetics. This is a scarring that occurs in the thick middle layer of your heart wall, which is the myocardium. Myocardial fibrosis is often due to the high blood glucose levels, which sets off damages and glycation of proteins in the myocardium.

Congestive heart failure is a heart problem where your heart does not pump enough blood to your body the energy it needs. You can take preventive steps to stop this problem before it starts.

Your heart is really a muscle that is a pump. The primary purpose is to circulate your blood which is about 2,000 gallons throughout your body. There are four chambers that are involved. You have two upper chambers which are the atria of the heart, and then there are the lower ones called ventricles. The ventricles are responsible for pumping your blood out properly. The valves of the heart separate the chambers. There are four valves that will open and close to send blood flowing properly through the body.

When you have CHF, your heart does not quit beating obviously. What happens though, is that the ventricles, sometimes both, or just one weaken and thus becomes unable to pump aggressively. This causes the blood flow to get behind and, as a result fluid will build up along with the blood with the heart not working properly. You will notice edema in parts of the body, (hands, and feet especially), and as the heart enlarges abnormally, it continues to become weaker over time. This is where failure comes in the heart.

People with diabetes are more likely to have CHF. Diabetes in and of itself is a high risk factor for various heart problems anyway.
The best way to prevent any future problems for developing CHF is by controlling your blood sugar levels, eating right, exercising, not smoking, and taking all insulins and medications as prescribed by your doctor.

Hypertension and Diabetes

Hypertension, (high blood pressure), is often linked with diabetes of each type 1 and 2. It plays a high risk factor for strokes, heart attacks, and kidney failure. High blood pressure is more common in diabetic people more than non-diabetic people. The cause of why this happens more often in diabetics is not really understood.

Hypertension is an aggravator for blood vessel damage already present in diabetics. High blood pressure is also the cause for more serious complications of diabetes including heart attacks, strokes, and kidney failure. This is why it is important to treat high blood pressure aggressively before it causes these problems.

Diabetics as well as non-diabetics need to keep their blood pressure at 130/80 or below. This blood pressure reading target greatly reduces the chances of stroke and heart attack happening.

Blood pressure is actually the action of the heart pumping blood more than 93 miles of blood vessels. This process acts like a plumbing system, transporting the blood to your vital organs. You need a certain amount of pressure going within this system to keep the blood flowing . But when there is too much pressure, it will damage the blood vessels and thus they become narrow.This is where serious health problems will occur.

A person's blood pressure is categorized in three ways. There is the normal, prehypertensive, or hypertensive. Stage 1 is the stage where blood pressure runs around 140/90 and up to 159/99. In stage 2, blood pressure is usually running around 160/100 or more. Blood pressure at that stage is very risky and needs to be treated as quickly as possible.

Your body has many ways of working with the blood pressure to be certain its organs, the brain especially, maintain the oxygen it needs to. Types of high blood pressure are divided into two groups. Group one is known to be essential or primary. This is the group that has no real known cause, and the most common form. Group two is defined as secondary high blood pressure. This group has a cause, and can sometimes be curable if the cause is able to be corrected.

The top number of the blood pressure is the systolic pressure and is measuring the force on the blood vessel walls as the heart is contracting. The second lower number, diastolic, is the force on the vessel walls as the heart is relaxing. Blood pressure measurement itself is known as millimeters of mercury, (mm Hg).

Many causes for primary hypertension are possible. The kidneys are number one. Kidneys have two main arteries, and when narrowed, the kidney transmits your blood pressure as being too low. The kidney then sends a signal out to raise the blood pressure, which causes hypertension. This is referred to by doctors as having renal artery hypertension. If the blocked artery to the kidney is opened, this usually corrects the problems.

Other causes for primary hypertension can be a possible thyroid problem you are having, and other hormonal factors. Contraceptives are also associated with high blood pressure, and smoking along with obesity is a problem that contributes to hypertensiveness.

So diabetics along with other non-diabetics should have their blood pressure taken on a regular basis. If you smoke, it really is best to quit since it does raise the blood pressure quite often. It is often known as the silent killer, and if left untreated, can lead to early death.

It is best to keep a blood pressure monitor at home so you can track your pressures on a daily basis. This helps you and your health care team to make the best treatment plan for you.

Article by David Cowley:

Understanding Your Blood Pressure Medication

There are many different types of blood pressure medications, and it's important that you understand what's been prescribed for you before you begin taking them. Some have serious side effects that you need to inform your doctor about, and others will cause drug interaction or allergic reactions if you do not communicate these things to your doctor as well. Most blood pressure medications work to slow your heartbeat, lessen the constriction of blood vessels, or cause your blood to become thinner. And while it's impossible to cover all the various medications and recommendations your doctor may give to you, we can give you some basic information about the most commonly prescribed blood pressure medications here:

Angiotensin

Angiotensin is an enzyme in the body that causes the blood vessels to constrict. Sometimes this is necessary, but too much of this element will cause them to become too narrow, which will necessitate your heart working harder to pump your blood through. Often a body produces too much of this enzyme, probably through genetics or simply imperfection of the circulatory system. Many blood pressure medications work to block this enzyme or the overproduction of it.

ACE inhibitors and ARB receptor blockers are two such blood pressure medications. By not allowing the overproduction of this enzyme, the blood vessels will not be overly constrictive and will allow the blood to flow much more freely.

Nitrates

Nitrates work by relaxing blood vessels throughout the entire body so that the heart, again, does not need to work as hard to pump the blood through. Nitrates are very common blood pressure medications. Some are not meant to be taken regularly but only when a patient feels the pain in the chest that happens when the heart is pumping too hard. These pills are often placed under the tongue in such emergencies. Some however will get nitrate pills, sprays, and even patches which will release this blood pressure medication in a regular dosage. This is important because this pain that signals the heart working too hard can be easily mistaken for indigestion or muscle cramps.

Vasodilators

These blood pressure medications work by causing the blood vessels to open up or dilate. Vasodilators are never used on a permanent basis or on their own, as eventually the kidneys would respond to these dilated blood vessels by retaining more water. It's important to be aware of the side effects of headache, rapid heart rate, and even sweating; if these become severe, you need to talk to your doctor. They can also cause fainting and dizziness, especially upon standing up.

Other blood pressure medications may include diuretics, which cause the body to lose water and therefore thin the blood, making it easier to push through the circulatory system, and beta blockers, which cause the heart to beat slower than normal. Whatever medication you've been prescribed, use it exactly as directed and tell your doctor of any side effects you're having.

Common Vitamins and over the counter products can help with heart disease such as Sytrinol, Policosanol, Potassium, Pectin, and M.S.M.

Sytrinol are known to be useful in helping maintain a healthy cholesterol level in the body by reducing triglycerides and low-density lipoprotein (LDL) levels.

Policosanol is a natural supplement derived from sugar cane. Policosanol promotes healthy platelet function and helps to maintain normal cholesterol levels in the human body.

Potassium is essential for proper functioning of the heart muscle and for regulating proper fluid balance. Bananas are a good source of potassium.

Pectin limits the amount of cholesterol the body can absorb. High pectin count in apples may be why "One a day keeps the doctor away".

M.S.M maintains the development of the body's protein by forming flexible disulfide bonds between certain amino acids and in maintaining the strength of connective tissue. This allows water and nutrients to flow freely into cells and allows toxins to flow freely out of the cells. M.S.M increases athletic stamina and helps eliminate muscle soreness. M.S.M is a natural supplement that is getting a lot of attention due to its role in tissue healing at the cellular level. It is a natural organic sulfur that comes from rainfall and is found naturally in the human body.

If you are at risk from Heart Disease then find a good health care professional prior to starting any type of home treatment.

Always consult your doctor before using this information.

Sexual Problems Related to Diabetes

The sexual problems of diabetes are related to nerve impulses or signals. The internal organs like the heart and bladder for example, are controlled by nerve signals as well. The body's response to sexual stimuli, would also be involuntary. Autonomic nerve signals increase the blood flow to the genitals and will cause smooth muscle tissue to relax. When the autonomic nerves are damaged, this will taper normal sexual functions.

Erectile Dysfunction Erectile dysfunction in men who have diabetes range from 20 to 85 percent. This problem is defined as the inability to have an erection, or the inability to sustain his erection.

Diabetic men are highly likely to have sexual problems concerning erectile dysfunction more than men who do not have diabetes. These diabetic men are also likely to have this problem much earlier than men without diabetes.

Other causes of erectile dysfunction include hypertension, kidney disease, alcoholism and blood vessel disease. ED may also occur because of medication and side effects, psychological factors, hormonal deficiencies, or smoking.

Men experiencing ED should talk to the doctor, which is step one in getting help. Your doctor should review your history with you, conduct lab tests, and other health problems you may have. There are also tests that you can do at home that checks for erections during sleeping time. Treatments for ED vary widely. Pills or a vacuum pump, pellets placed in the urethra, or shots may be recommended.

Retrograde Ejaculation Retrograde ejaculation is known as a sexual problem where all or part of a man's semen goes into the bladder instead of out the penis during ejaculation. Retrograde ejaculation happens when muscles which are internal called sphincters will not function properly. The sphincter should automatically open or close a passage in the body. Semen combines urine in the bladder and leaves the body during urination, without harmful effects to the bladder. When a man experiences retrograde ejaculation, he may notice that little semen is discharged during ejaculation. The urine will appear cloudy chances are, and urinalysis will reveal the presence of semen. Blood sugars not controlled and the nerve damage due to this, are associated with retrograde ejaculation. Another reason for retrograde ejaculation might be prostate surgery or hypertensive medications.

Medication can be prescribed for retrograde ejaculation caused by diabetes. Most urologists experienced in the fields of fertility treatments can have ways to promote fertility.

Decreased Vaginal Lubrication Vaginal dryness in women often results from nerve damage to cells inside the vaginal area. This leads to great pain during sexual activity. As a result, this leads to lesser sexual responses.

Decreased or Absent Sexual Response Sexual problems caused by diabetes, blood pressure pills, and certain other prescribed medicines, drug or alcohol abuse can contribute to a diminished sexual response. An infection of a gynecologic nature, or conditions that relate to being pregnant or menopause, also do not help a woman's sexuality.
As many as 35-40 percent of women that are diabetic may have decreased or lack of interest in sex. As a result, the ability to achieve orgasm will probably result. Symptoms of a woman's sexual problems include the following:

No interest in sex.
A decrease or no sensations in the genital area.
No orgasm.The inability to achieve an orgasm.
Dryness in the vaginal area that is painful during sexual relations.

If you as a woman have any problems sexually, speak to your doctor and go over your complete history thoroughly. As with men, lab tests will usually be performed to help sort out the causes for these problems. Sometimes prescriptions or over-the-counter vaginal creams that serve as a lubricant may be helpful for ladies having a problem with dryness. Counseling is sometimes in order as well as Kegel exercises that strengthen bladder muscles may be helpful too.

Vaginal Yeast Infections and Diabetes

Vaginal yeast infections and diabetes can be a frequent problem for diabetic females. Candidus is the most common infection type, and it is hard to get rid of. When a female has repetitive yeast infections, and is not aware of diabetes as a possible cause, it is best to have a fasting blood sugar test and find out. All of us have a certain balance of both good and bad bacteria within our bodies, which we need to have. Bad bacteria, believe it or not, is a necessity, but only within limits. When the bad bacteria goes beyond certain levels. we become ill, such as with vaginal candida related yeast infections.

A diabetic has to work harder to have a stronger immune system than non-diabetics. We as diabetics have to stay within certain healthy levels so that we don't create an imbalance by watching our diet, taking insulin shots and medications as prescribed, and also exercising. Being aware of the symptoms of candida infection is important, as it does take longer to get rid of as a diabetic person.

The one main symptom vaginal yeast infections, (any yeast infection), is an intense miserable vaginal itching. There will probably also be a vaginal discharge. You may also feel very unwell.

The reason diabetic women have this problem so much more frequently, is the blood sugar levels being unstable, which throws off the body chemistry and causes these irritating infections.

There are many treatment options available for diabetics and for yeast infections. Monistat works really well and Vagisil alleviates a lot of the troublesome itching. But you may also need a doctor to prescribe medications to rid your body of the problem. Sexual activity does not help vaginal yeast infections. Use protection during sex to not aggra-vate the problem.

Sick Days with Your Diabetes

Dealing with sick days when a person has colds, flus, and other illnesses are difficult for people without diabetes. But for those of us with diabetes, we need a lot of special self-care and maybe even a doctor visit.

First of all, when you are sick with colds and flu as a diabetic, your blood sugars usually go up sky high. This can lead to other complications that can put you in a comatose state. Working out a plan for sick days ahead of time is best. You can devise a plan of what to do, and have the supplies on hand just in case.

Your body under stress with illness and diabetes. To deal with the stresses of cold or flu, you body automatically releases hormones that are working to fight it off. The hormones have side effects however, which is raising blood glucose levels that interfere with your injected insulin. If taking diabetes pills, they lose their effectiveness during this time, and the result of high sugars happen as well in this case.

Type 1 diabetics may develop serious ketoacidosis leading to coma. And those of us with type 2 diabetes can develop something referred to as hyperosmolar hyperglycemic nonketotic coma, where just like in type 1, the blood sugars go out of sight. These conditions are both dangerous and very life-threatening. But a lot of times you can avoid this by following your sick days plan.

Working with your doctor or health care team on a sick day plan is really important. The plan should include in it, what to do if you need to call on your team for more help. You should also keep your plan somewhere handy so you can reach help right away.

For minor illnesses, you probably won't need to consult your doctor. But if these things listed happens, it is time to pick up the phone for help:

You can't shake a fever.
You keep on vomiting or having diarrhea all day.
You are seeing ketones on a urine test.
Your blood sugar will not go down from very high, which means 180 or more.
You are on diabetes pills and your sugars keep going up.
You cannot hold liquids at all and are becoming steadily dehydrated. Very dangerous very any diabetic.
You have other symptoms of illness you are unsure of and don't know what to do.

When you see the doctor, take medications with you including the over-the-counter drugs. They are equally important along with prescribed medications. Tell your doctor how long you have been sick and what is going on if you are unable to hold anything down.

Eating and drinking can be problematic when you are ill. You need to stick with your meal plan if able to. If not, here are some good sick day eating ideas:

1 cup warm diet soda Cold soda will agitate an upset stomach.
Soda crackers.
Dry toast
Hot plain broth eaten slowly
Sugar-free pudding
Mashed potatoes
1/2 cup Jello

Over the counter medicines may help you feel better as well, but do be careful and consult with your doctor's office on which ones are okay for a diabetic. This is very important in keeping away from unpleasant side effects leading to complications.

The key is staying in control of your blood glucose and getting the rest your body needs to heal properly. Sleeping extra is also a wonderful form of therapy and I think helps the body heal faster.

If your illness is severe enough to go to the ER, please take all of your medical information with you on your diabetes care. This is very important as I well know, when you see a doctor not familiar with you.

Hospitalization happens to most everyone at some point in their lives or another.

And while hospitalized, your diabetes care regime may differ greatly from what you do at home in your daily management.

When you are admitted into the hospital, you need to make certain that your doctor and the nurses caring for you understand your routine, medications and insulin, and how you manage it at home. Achieving the best care possible is important while there.

Being an inpatient is stressful enough with worrying about why you are there in the first place. An illness in your body stresses you out, along with surgeries you may be having, and other medical tests. Your routine care in hospitalization should include regular blood sugar monitoring by the nurses. Results should be noted in your hospital chart. Insulin and medication doses should be timed properly with meals and there should be the right dosages made according to your glucose testing results.

Your admitting doctor should also be looking at your needs for possible medication and insulin adjustments. A lot of your hospitals have their own standards of high or low blood sugar levels which may differ from your standards at home. If your blood sugar drops drastically while in the hospital, it should be treated promptly.

The hospital typically gives insulin to most diabetic patients. Insulin will either be given intravenously or by injection. If you are on a pump, short acting insulin may be prescribed.

Insulin given by IV is usually given if you are having surgery, which creates a lot more stress on the body, then for a non-diabetic. If you are on steroidal drugs, having cardiac problems, have ketoacidosis and dehydration, the intravenous insulin will definitely be called for.

Glucose monitoring is an important factor while in the hospital. This helps the hospital staff and your doctor keep strict tabs on your glucose control. The blood sugar monitoring in the hospital is just like you do it at home. The only thing different is they use their own Accu-chek meter instead of yours. Your glucose tracking by medical people there will be tailored to your individual needs. Most frequently, it is done about every 4-6 hours.

Your diabetic meal plan in the hospital will usually consist of a balanced carbohydrate meal plan. If you are scheduled for surgery, then liquids served instead will contain sufficient carbohydrate such as clear broth. The carbohydrate is needed before surgery to prevent some serious hypoglycemia. Before you leave the hospital, a nutritionist or dietitian should give you a good meal plan that will fit your needs at home while you are recovering from whatever surgery or illnesses you have.

Above all, you need to speak up for yourself if you don't understand something that the hospital personnel is doing differently other than what you do at home. Don't be afraid to question anyone, or talk with your doctor about your care during the hospital stay. Your health is very important with diabetes, and achieving the best control of blood sugar during this time is of the utmost importance.

Pernicious Anemia

Pernicious anemia is a type of anemia where there is a vitamin B12 deficiency. It is sometimes seen in a type 1 diabetic since this is classified as an autoimmune disorder.

In the body's immune system, there is sometimes an attack on the parietal cells in the stomach. This is how this type of anemia is often caused. The parietal cells make a protein called intrinsic factor, which is the body's helper in absorbing vitamin B12. Thus, when these parietal cells become destroyed, the B12 vitamins will not be absorbed in the correct way they should be. Then the lack of the B12 keeps the red blood cells from dividing normally, causing them to become too large.

What happens next is that these cells have trouble leaving the bone marrow. You also need B12 for your nervous system to work in the right way.

Pernicious anemia is a big cause for other medical problems throughout the body. When a person has this type of anemia, the heart has to work a lot harder in order to pump enough blood for nourishments to the tissues inside the body. The heart then, begins to have arrhythmias, and fast beats. This in turn can lead to heart attacks and even strokes. Damage to the nervous system causes other things like numbness, and tingling in both hands and feet. There can be difficulty with keeping your balance, visual changes, memory loss, and mental confusion. Other symptomatology can include loss of appetite, diarrhea, and fatigue.

The good news is that pernicious anemia is easily treatable with B12 injections. There are people though that sometimes develop some permanent damage in the nerves before they are diagnosed. But if caught early, damages are unlikely to happen.

There are several other autoimmune diseases that can happen in combination because type 1 is an autoimmune disease and a trigger for these problems. Thyroiditis is also in that category of autoimmune problems along with Graves disease. I will do more articles on these problems and put links to them on this page so that people may learn how they tie in to diabetes.

Pregnancy and Diabetes

Pregnancy and diabetes takes some sensible planning as a diabetic woman. You will need to have tight blood glucose control, as hyperglycemia during pregnancy can pose risks to the unborn baby. There are other risks involved with pregnancy and diabetes, like spontaneous abortions, miscarriages, or ectopic pregnancies in women with diabetes. There are also chances of the baby becoming very big, making it a difficult birth. And a difficult birth poses problems for the newborn child such as hypoglycemia.

When diabetic females become pregnant, they need to have clear target blood glucose ranges in mind. Blood sugar levels should be kept at something like:

70-100 Fasting and before meals
Below 140 1 hour after meals
Below 120 2 hours after meals

Your healthcare team in your pregnancy should be well-rounded and include a dietitian, endocrinologist, your regular MD, and of course your obstetrician. Your team during pregnancy should coordinate and work together to serve your healthcare needs during this time.

Prenatal vitamins are also strongly advised in diabetes and pregnancy, as for women who are not diabetic. Vitamin B with folic acid is important to lower the risks of birth defects with the unborn baby.
If you are having any diabetes complications, it can make diabetes and pregnancy very risky. Anything like retinopathies, kidney problems you are having, or other related diabetic problems will have to be monitored very closely while pregnant. You will need to be carefully treated closely to avoid any serious problems happening with yourself and the baby. Some women decide after having diabetic problems that it is often not worth becoming pregnant as it can carry serious risks.

Children born from diabetic women also have a higher risk of coming down with diabetes themselves. When a woman has type 1 diabetes, her offspring have about a 5% chance of developing diabetes in their lifetimes. When the male and female both have diabetes of type 1 or 2, chances are very high that the offspring will develop diabetes sometime in their life, about 40%.

Overall, women that decide to become pregnant with diabetes and have the very best care, have much lower chances of having children with a birth defect.

For good books on pregnancy and diabetes care, I suggest reading Diabetes and Pregnancy: What to Expect, 4th Edition. This is an excellent source of advice of all the best things to do while expecting children. Another one is 101 Tips for a Healthy Pregnancy with Diabetes. Either of these can be found at Amazon.com.

Breastfeeding Moms with Diabetes

Breastfeeding moms with diabetes are helping their infant's health.

There have been certain studies done that actually prove breastfeeding moms can help their newborn baby to prevent type 1 diabetes. Breastfeeding for at least a 6 month period up to one year sure very positive effects to these children as they grow.

It has been maintained that the nutrients in breast milk which is the colostrum promote a steady growth rate in babies unlike those who have received formulas instead.

Other benefits to nursing your newborn baby help you lose weight from the pregnancy, and this is important for women with diabetes. Women nursing their babies also find it easier to manage their blood glucose levels since they have a remission of some symptoms in nursing their newborns.

Blood sugar monitoring is important during this period of time. You may find out that your sugars are more stable, and therefore the needs for insulin levels lower. The insulin does not get into your child's body. This is simply because it is too big to get into your milk. If you are only on diabetes pills however, you need to be on a medicine that will not get ingested by the baby.

Watching your diet is important while nursing. Snacking is beneficial during this time since you need to keep your blood sugar levels steady. Increasing the amounts of calories you take in is also important for the reasons of your child's nourishment. Drinking a can of Ensure will give you the vitamins and minerals you and the baby need.

Your diet also needs proper balancing. You need at least 30-40% from fruits and vegetables, and also 40-60% from protein sources. Do not forget to include at least 40-60% in carbohydrates especially whole grain sources which are best. Be aware of hypoglycemia. This is why you need to track blood sugars closely over this period. You need to include plenty of legumes in your diet as well. Fluids are equally important as healthy solid foods. You need to stay as healthy as possible with your newborn baby.

After your child is delivered, breastfeeding right away is an important thing to do to avoid a hypoglycemic situation. Nurses many times will take the child away for examinations. But you can insist as a breastfeeding mom that the baby remain with you for nursing purposes, and also getting to know your child.

When you are diabetic, your milk may come in later than nondiabetic women. Sometimes it can take anywhere from three, four days, and as long as two weeks. A breast pump can help this problem and the baby will still receive all of the nutrients from the milk that they need.

Gestational Diabetes

Gestational diabetes is produced sometimes occurs in women right about the 26th or more week of pregnancy. What causes gestational diabetes is not exactly known, but some ideas have been found. The baby gets its support from the placenta which helps the child develop properly. Those hormones from the placenta though, also block the action of the woman's insulin in her body. This problem is defined as insulin resistance. The insulin resistance makes it very difficult to use insulin. This means then, that a pregnant woman may need up to three times as much insulin than normal.

Gestational diabetes will start if your body is unable to produce and use the insulin it needs for pregnancy. And when you don't have enough insulin, the blood sugar cannot leave the blood and be used for energy as it should. The blood sugar then keeps building up in your blood to high levels. It is then labeled as hyperglycemia.

This type of diabetes does not cause the types of birth defects seen in babies where the woman has had diabetes before pregnancy.If this diabetes is not under control during the pregnancy period, however, it can hurt the baby.The reason being is that your pancreas when pregnant works overtime to produce insulin. And whatever insulin **does not** lower your blood sugar or cross the placenta. Extra blood sugars then get into the placenta, giving the baby high blood sugar levels. The baby's pancreas is made to produce extra insulin to get rid of the blood glucose. With the baby getting more energy than it needs to grow and develop, that extra energy is stored as fat.

This process in turn, can lead to a fat baby. Babies that are born overweight face potential health problems of their own. And then because of the extra insulin made by the baby's pancreas, infants may experience hypoglycemia, (low blood sugars), at birth, and therefore at higher risk for breathing problems.Babies can also be at risk for obesity and adults geared toward type 2 diabetes.

To treat this form of diabetes since it can hurt you and your baby, you need treatment immediately. The treatment goal is to keep blood sugar levels like other women who do not have this diabetic problem. Treatment also includes meal plans low in carbs, and exercise as you are able, even light activity. Frequent doctor visits are necessary, and glucose testing at home too.

Smoking and Diabetes

Smoking and diabetes is a deadly combination. It is the most addictive of habits once started, and the biggest cause of death. Many cancers arise from smoking such as lung, mouth, and even pancreatic cancers. Diabetics who smoke need to learn how to overcome addiction to nicotine fast before it makes their condition any worse.

When a person has diabetes though, many more health problems can arise very easily. Here are some things that can happen to the diabetic person:

Blood flow problems Diabetes causes blood flow problems many times anyway. But with the use of cigarettes, the blood flow will be cut down even more.

Sexual problems Diabetes often causes erectile dysfunction in men, but cigarettes most definitely will compound this problem along with other sexual problems.

High Cholesterol Diabetes, especially in type 2, can cause abnormal levels of high bad (LDL, cholesterol as well as atherosclerosis, which is a hardening of the arteries. This is another problem with smoking and diabetes.

Heart Disease which is common with a diabetic person many times. Smoking will surely promote this problem even more so.

Oxygen Cigarettes harm the amount of oxygen you have that gets into your tissues. These can lead to heart attacks, strokes, miscarriages, and babies born dead.

Respiratory problems are more common when using cigarettes. Since it is irritating to the lungs, colds and upper respiratory infections happen much quicker.

Joint problems are promoted when you smoke, and especially with diabetes. Diabetes can cause a number of bone problems as pointed out within this site many times. Smoking compounds these problems and causes limited mobility all the more.

Hypertension is a common problem when a person smokes. The nicotine in cigarettes automatically raise the blood pressure. Diabetes makes a person at risk for hypertension anyway, but by smoking, this is a hypertension invitation for sure.

Glucose levels are raised by cigarettes. Nicotine has a way of doing this especially with someone who is already diabetic. This makes your diabetic situation hard to manage every day.

Heart attacks are compounded when you add smoking and diabetes to the mix. This is a sure way to introduce heart disease to your body which is already trying to normalize blood sugars.

Smoking is hard to quit **since the nicotine is very very addictive to a person. In quitting smoking, there are withdrawal symptoms such as restlessness, dizziness, headaches, sweating,** and having diarrhea. But by hanging in there, these things will go away over a period of time once the body is no longer used to having nicotine addiction.

Author Mike Tannen shares his thoughts on smoking:

How to Get 80% of Your Body Destroyed

Imagine your body as a bustling city, smoking cigarette with its 3,000 chemical components will be just like a fleet of bombers setting off to carpet bomb it - with your permission. Smoking harms nearly every organs in the body, and while the theory of each cigarette reducing 11.5 minutes of your life may not be completely true (some smokers live up to their 90s), it's almost certain that in near future you will be spending over 85% of your pension fund undoing smoking damages. Now did you just mention about happy retirement?

Let's start the journey from head to feet; in the head smoking speeds up brain decline, five times faster than non-smokers. Carbon monoxide deprives your brain of oxygen - this blurred a person's ability to accurately judge their actions in long term. Next would be mouth or throat cancer, which 90% of sufferers are smokers; just think of having persistent sore throat, nose inflammation, swollen lymph glands in the neck, sticky phlegm coughs, total loss of voice, or traces of blood in saliva. Life would be dreadful isn't it?

The greatest visible impact will be on your teeth. Tar is responsible for staining your teeth, yellowing it to an unpleasant extent, and this can only be removed with professional dental cleaning. In the meantime, smoking also weakens your gums and caused bad breath. Your non-smoker friends and work colleagues may look at you as someone who doesn't have tooth brushing habit.

Widely documented as the most harmful smoking effects, the lungs absorbed almost everything from a cigarette. Every time you smoke, a portion of air sacks in your lungs (Alveoli) is killed. They won't grow back, which means you have permanently destroyed part of your lungs.

The little hair-like structures that help sweep particles out of your lungs (Cilia) are also paralyzed by smoke. Now that the lungs auto-cleaning mechanisms are gone, tar from the cigarette can safely be coated throughout your lungs, blacken it, and eventually causes cancer.

The heart too, is not immune to the effects of smoking. Carbon monoxide in the cigarette smoke increases the amount of cholesterol and constricts blood vessels. This is harmful as it clogs up heart arteries and may lead to heart failure one day. Your heart will now need to work extra hard to pump the same amount of blood as it used to in the past. The thousands of chemicals you smoke in will now dissolve into the blood and be pumped by the heart to everywhere in the body, with consequences that will be detailed below.

Human biology is quite simple, all organs in the body need oxygen, and they are dependent on the heart to pump oxygenated blood for them. But when the heart pumps blood with something else in it, things won't just go normal. The skin, as the largest organ, will be the first to be affected. Poor blood circulation and a partial loss of oxygen will cause premature aging and wrinkles to form; you will look more aged than your actual age.

Reduced oxygen supply also weakens bones, joints and muscles, hence increased chances of fractures and tissue injuries. When tar finally reaches your kidney and colon, it doesn't get flushed out as waste, instead depositing itself there. This is disastrous as you cannot clean them out like how you clean dirt off your car, and it will eventually grow cancerous.

Having learnt so many harmful smoking effects, one of the questions most smokers may ask "With so much damage already done, what's the use I quit now?" Well don't give up, your inner biology returns to its normal state in just 3 months after quitting, and your risk of cancer will resume to nearly the same level as people who have never smoked after several years - so it isn't really too late. quit smoking now, your body has tried its best everyday to puff out all those harmful chemicals you installed onto it, why ruin its efforts?

Get ready to quit smoking? Ridding the harmful smoking effects all at once? Now here is the good news; you don't need nicotine patches, gums, some 'cold turkey' method, or even try to cope with the withdrawal syndrome.

Diabetes and Your Oral Health
Dental health and your diabetes are very important in keeping away complications. Diabetes is often a cause for periodontal or gum disease. Your immune system is often weakened by diabetes, and this is a nest for problems. As a result of this problem, your mouth is the target area for bleeding gums, and as a result germs begin multiplying there.

These germs promote periodontal disease because they make a substance which will alter the way the cells process carbohydrates in the body. There are many research studies that also demonstrate that bacteria causes high blood glucose levels and also more insulin resistance.

When your diabetes is out of control, it can really raise havoc with dental hygiene. When your blood sugars are high, it results in lack of saliva in your mouth. Therefore what happens is you have trouble with processing salivary sugars. This can then lead to mouth ulcers, which create bigger problems. So this explains why keeping your blood sugars in control, plays a big role in helping to control diabetes, and keeping a healthy mouth free from periodontal disease.

Are you not happy with your current smile? Visit the best San Diego orthodontist to transform your smile.

For your diabetes and dental health, flossing your teeth is also very important along with brushing three times daily. Your oral hygiene is essential to also preventing tooth decaying, and also losing teeth. There are a certain amount of circulatory problems that go along with diabetes, and this does not help your oral care. That is why it is extremely important to protect your teeth all you can, avoiding another area of complications along the way.

Brushing and flossing is a very important part of keeping better oral hygiene and protecting yourself against major mouth problems and advance dental disease.

Frozen shoulder

Frozen shoulder, typically known as adhesive capsulitis. This means that your shoulder is totally stiff. The shoulder becomes impossible to move around, and doing even simple tasks is painful.

In the beginning of this problem, your shoulder will definitely pain you a lot. Therefore when this happens, you don't move it around or at all. And with not moving it around, your joints will stiffen up all the more.
As your shoulder gradually becomes stiffer, you use it even less and are afraid to even move it a tiny bit. What happens then? You lose range of motion of course, and it won't budge anyhow due to pain and even greater stiffness.
A frozen shoulder can happen due to an injury, or a bout with another bone problem such as bursitis, or tendonitis.

How does diabetes connect with a frozen shoulder? Well, one theory involves collagen, which is one of your main sources of ligaments and tendons. Collagen holds the bones together since it is holding bones together in joints. When glucose rises, it affects collagen, which is deposited abnormally into the tendons and cartilage of your shoulder. This buildup over time, causes you to lose range of motion, and your shoulder then stiffens up.

This problem affects about 30 percent of diabetic people, in comparison to only 7 percent of people who are nondiabetic.
This particular problem in the joints of the shoulder comes up in stages. You will notice pains at first, which is a generalized aching. There could even be spasms in the muscles.
The next thing to happen is maybe not quite so painful, but more inflexible, lack of motion, and stiffness. This second stage can go on for maybe six months at the most.

The third stage is the stage of recovery. As in stage one, this stage is not as painful. Your shoulder and arm might regain some or most of the neutral movement as the ligaments begin to stretch. The recovery may be off and on, with some painfulness as the lining of joints stretch out.

Treating frozen shoulder early is important to keep the shoulder moving and with a range of motion still. Physical therapies may help, even though there is pain. The lack of use only makes the problem worse, and this is why therapy helps, though yes, it's painful.

Motrin and Ibuprofen are great pain helpers, and will help a person start therapy. Your therapist will generally work with you, seeing how your tolerance for movement is, and going from there.

If there is more severe pain on the other hand from this problem, you should work with your doctor to find relief from either shots or oral medications that can be prescribed.

With pain that is only mild, and not too intense in your joints, you can try moist heat, Ibuprofen or Motrin for a little while. However, when your arm movements get so you can't move it at all, you need to see your doctor for treatment.

Surgery is also another option for this problem if need be, and it is intolerable to live with. It should be the very last thing to consider, but

Trigger finger, commonly known as stiff hand syndrome, is a frequent occurrence in people with diabetes.

It is actually more frequent in long-standing type 1 diabetes. But type 2 diabetics have been known to experience this problem just as well. Diabetes will often target hands as a good place for more complications, and stiff-hand syndrome is one of them along with carpal-tunnel syndrome.

Range of motion in the joints is limited as it is in frozen shoulder.

What you will notice with stiff-hand syndrome, is that your hand will have limited mobility in it. A thick, tight, waxy skin is part of the symptomatology of this disorder.

The cause of this problem has been linked to increased glycosylation of collagen in the skin, and also diabetic neuropathy. Contractures of the fingers known as flexion, may develop when the problem reaches advanced stages.

One of the signs most noticeable with trigger finger is the formation of the prayer sign. When a person is unable to completely close gaps between palms together, this is an indicator of stiff-hand syndrome. Also, many people complain of a locking or catching sensation accompanied by pain in the fingers.

Corticosteroids may help this condition along with some physical therapy. Ibuprofen or Motrin also can kill the pain associated with this problem.

Dr. Francois L Botha shares his perspective:

Frozen shoulder is a common condition that affects many people. In the medical world frozen shoulder is known as adhesive capsulitis. The main symptoms of frozen shoulder are both pain and stiffness in the shoulder joint. It is quite common for a person to be suffering from this condition in one shoulder but not the other.

There is one stage of this condition that you should be most concerned with; this is called the frozen stage. It is during this time that you will notice the decreased range of motion in the affected shoulder. For most people this is when it is necessary to see a doctor.

Unfortunately, doctors do not know the exact cause of frozen shoulder. Most commonly, frozen shoulder occurs in people who have not used the joint for an extended period of time. This is common among people who have had surgery or a broken bone in the arm. But with that being said, frozen shoulder can happen for many other unexplained reasons as well.

Frozen shoulder is a result of the shoulder capsule becoming inflamed for one reason or the next. In turn, tissue can build up between the surface of the joints and this can lead to extreme pain and lost range of motion. In the most severe cases frozen shoulder can affect movement so much that even day to day tasks are seemingly impossible.

If you feel that you may be suffering from frozen shoulder you will want to consult with your doctor right away. They will be able to give you the proper diagnose, and then provide you with the necessary level of treatment. The most common treatment methods include anti-inflammatory drugs, heat or cold compresses, shoulder manipulation, and in the most severe cases surgery.

Frozen shoulder can be quite bothersome regardless of the level of activity that you take part in. Luckily, there are plenty of treatment options that you can consider if your frozen shoulder has gotten too far out of control. Remember, your best bet is to consult with a doctor in order to get the proper diagnosis.

Treatment Options for Frozen Shoulder

Moist heat has been found very effective for frozen shoulder pain. Just take a heat pad and put a moist towel under it, and apply both to your shoulder.

Ice can help with frozen shoulder pain as well. To be the most effective, put your ice on for 10 minutes on your shoulder, and 10 minutes off. You can also alternate ice and moist heat.

Physical therapy has also helped with the pain of frozen shoulder. If you think this would help, ask your doctor to give you a referral for a good physical therapist.

Although anti-inflammatory medications haven't helped change the course of a frozen shoulder, they can give substantial relief from the painful symptoms.

Your doctor may suggest one or more cortisone injections. These injections can really help to decrease pain, and in also let you stretch more. This is very important, because it's usually only effective when used together with physical therapy.

If all else fails, a surgeon may perform what's called a manipulation. A manipulation is done with the patient sedated, and the doctor moves the arm to break up adhesions caused by frozen shoulder. There are no incisions made during the procedure.

This next set of tips will give you some great stretches and exercises that you can do to help relieve and treat your frozen shoulder.

This exercise you can do while standing or sitting. Hold a 5- to 10-pound weight in your hand (a gallon of water or milk weighs 8 pounds) and keep your arm vertical and close to your body. Swing your arm back and forth or in a small diameter circle.

For this exercise, put your arm onto a shelf or a dresser about breast high. Gently bend your knees, and open your arm pit. Try to push the arm up a little farther with each stretch.

For this exercise, take a bath towel and hold it with both hands at a 45 degree angle. Use your good arm to pull the towel toward your lower back. You can repeat this with your towel in a horizontal position.

To do this exercise, face a wall about 18 inches away. Using your fingers instead of your shoulder muscles, raise your arm up to shoulder level. Repeat this 5-10 times.

Grab a rubber band for these next few exercises. For this one, hold your elbows at 90 degrees, close to your sides. Grab the rubber band with both hands, and turn your forearms outward only two or three inches, holding for five seconds. Do this 5-10 times.

For this one, arms the same way as the previous exercise. Hook your rubber band onto a door handle and hold it with one hand. Turn your forearm inward two or three inches (like a door), and hold it for five seconds. Do this 3-5 times.

Here's another fun exercise you can do with a rubber band. Bend your elbow again, and place the rubber band on a door like before. Lift your arm up four or five inches away from the body (like lifting weights), holding for five seconds. Repeat this 3-5 times.

You can do this exercise while watching TV or sitting at a traffic light. Simply shrug your affected shoulder up and down slowly 5-10 times a day.

This is an exercise that you've probably done as a kid, but it can help with your frozen shoulder. Simply hold your arm out, and make circles with it. Take turns making small and large circles.

It's a bit unconventional, but some people find that leg stretches can really help with frozen shoulder. For this exercise, lay down on your back in front of a doorway. Put one leg up the wall and one leg out flat, with your arms resting at your side. This pose is good for stretching the hamstrings of one leg and the hip flexors of the other. Hold it for 2-5 minutes.

If you're having trouble sleeping at night, try using an extra pillow. Put the pillow under your affected shoulder, and sleep on your back or side.

Massage has helped many people with frozen shoulder. The muscles surrounding your frozen shoulder can become sore and tired. Massage can help alleviate these sore muscles.

Here are some supplements that have been known to help with frozen shoulder:

Glucosamine
Fish Oil
Honey Bee Venom

TENS stands for Transcutaneous Electrical Nerve Stimulation. It's a good and safe way to help with pain and relax muscles. It works by stimulating the skin nerves, thus helps the brain to ignore incoming pain signals from the joint.

Trigger point therapy is a type of specialized self massage that weeds out and removes painful muscular contractions. It works by applying pressure to the contractions, either with your fingers or massage tools.

Yoga is for straightening out your whole body, and it can really help with frozen shoulder. If you want to try yoga, start out slow and easy. If it winds up causing you more pain, yoga probably isn't for you.

A common mistake of people with frozen shoulder is that they keep it still. This is not always the best thing to do. Gentle movement will help to keep the blood flowing to your shoulder.

If you don't have frozen shoulder but are worried about risk factors, the best way to prevent it is by doing daily stretches. Refer to the stretches and exercise section of this ebook for ideas.

Like every health condition or ailment, new research and studies are being done every day to better help you cope with frozen shoulder. Use the internet and any other sources available to you to inform yourself of new treatments.

Traveling with Diabetes

Traveling with diabetes can be a challenge, and does take some real planning when going on vacations. You need to plan carefully well ahead of time, and gather all of your necessities together.
The first thing to think about is how you manage your glucose at home. You need to use this same plan when traveling, gathering all of your supplies together, and making certain to take your medicines and/or insulin at the right times. When going away from home, everything does change, especially the timing of meals, and the amount of activities you are doing.

First on your list, should be to make sure you have plenty of medications and insulins on hand so that you don't run out. If going on the airplane, it is best to have medicines and insulins in your carry on, as well as in your baggage. Luggage gets lost all the time in airports. And if you are insulin-dependent using syringes and not pumps, this could be a very tough situation. So that is why it is wise to have medicines and insulins in two places. Better to be safe then sorry!

Always carry coolers for insulin. If insulin gets hot, you will not be able to use it and injecting it anyhow, will make you very sick. Check your diabetic supply place or drugstore for a cooler that will keep your insulin nice and cold for protection against hot climates.

If you are taking a trip outside the US, do your homework first and find out where medical help is available in the country you are traveling to. Also check out if airlift is available in that country should a big emergency arise, and whether insurance covers it.

Have extra copies of prescriptions available in the rare case that you have forgotten to bring something. Always keep these extra scripts in your carry-on bags or purse. That way, it can easily be filled if you need it.

Above all, you need to carry these essential items traveling with diabetes:
Your doctor's phone number for emergencies
Your blood sugar meter
If you have a pump, you'll need syringes in case the pump quits!
A supply of glucose tablets should always be there.
Little snacks like granola bars or whole-grain crackers.
Glucagon is important if you tend to have severe lows from short acting insulin shots.
Ketone test strips for Type 1 diabetics.
A back-up pump. Some companies will loan you one for extra travel in case something happens to your current pump.

Even though trips are a challenge with diabetes, having everything you need is essential in order to have a safe trip without incidents. Always be sure you plan well ahead!

Strokes and Diabetes

Strokes are common in people with diabetes that have trouble in controlling their glucose levels.

These brain events are commonly known as a cerebrovascular accident. This happens when the blood supply to part of the brain becomes interrupted, causing brain cells to die within minutes. The damages to the brain can continue for many days after you have had this medical emergency.

These traumatic brain events are one of the leading causes of death in the US, and affects at least 650,000 people each year. People that have diabetes are much more likely to have a brain-related event then non-diabetic people.

Having a stroke is a medical emergency. The quicker medical attention is received, the better for the person to make a fuller recovery. Waiting to receive quick treatment can result in more brain damage occurring in brain tissue. This means a loss of speech or paralysis, and sometimes death can occur. There are two types of events concerning stroke:

Ischemic brain event. This is the most common medical emergency which is brought on by the lack of blood supply into the brain. There are two causes known for this event, and that is blood clots forming inside the artery because of atherosclerosis, or it can travel right through the bloodstream from another part of the body and lodges itself inside an artery known as an embolus. These conditions are termed as thrombotic and embolic stroke.

Hemorrhagic events are the type that occurs when blood from the arteries leaks out into the brain after a rupture has taken place. Besides starving the brain of essential blood and oxygen needed, the blood that has accumulated can cause more damage by exerting pressure on the brain in the surrounding tissue. Bleeding from in the brain (called cerebral hemorrhaging), accounts for a small percentage of strokes.

Bleeding around the brain which is subarachnoid hemorrhaging, accounts for an even smaller still, percentage of these medical events, like around 3%. Hemorrhaging cerebrally is usually brought on by hypertension, which according to what I've read, affects 70-75 percent of diabetics. A subarachnoid hemorrhaging event could also come from a ruptured aneurysm, which is when the arterial wall is bulging out. Head injuries can also bring on these traumatic brain events.

Type 1 diabetics have a higher risk of a major brain event since high blood glucose does damage the blood vessels over time. This makes the arterial walls thicker and less flexible, and prevents passage of blood. Type 2 diabetics are just as much at risk. Diabetics with type 1 or 2, tend to have a higher level of fats, especially type 2. This narrows and clogs blood vessels that result in atherosclerosis. People with diabetes are more prone to blood clots therefore, more than non-diabetics.

Diabetics are more likely as well to have coronary artery disease, obesity, and many other risk factors that bring on strokes.
The best way for diabetics to guard themselves from a serious brain event is by taking one aspirin a day unless you have very thin blood or bleeding problems, watching blood pressure, as well as taking control
of your diabetes and exercising.

Diabetes and Aneurysms come in different types. Diabetes can cause this complication along with strokes.

Though the brain is the most common area there are also:

Peripheral types that occur within the arteries. These can occur in the back of the thigh in the knee area. The area of the groin is another location as well as the carotid artery. These are not likely to rupture, although clots can form and block blood flow.

Diabetes and Aneurysms Symptoms

Abdominal types are the ones that slowly develop over a period of several years. This is another problem Doctors can sometimes tell when they feel a pulsating mass on examinations. The signs of this can also include:

A penetrating pain that is deep in the back or on the abdomen side.

A pain in your abdomen that will go on for many hours or weeks.

You may have a feeling that is either cold or numb. There may also be a tingling in the feet. This is due to the blood flow that has trouble reaching where it should in the lower extremities.

Cerebral Aneurysms

Cerebral aneurysms are those that happen in a brain artery. These are often silent, and when ready to rupture, give a warning sign of a severe headache. This is the main symptom. They will cause a stroke after rupturing, and easily lead to death. And with diabetes and aneurysms, they need to be looked at quickly or death can result.

Vomiting
Stiffness in the neck

If you are having any of these symptoms, it is wise to seek medical treatment quickly where you can get help quickly. Women have more chances of a cerebral occurrence than men.

Thoracic Aneurysms
These are the types in the chest that also have no symptoms with them unless the affected area begins to leak or grow. You might have:

Jaw pain

Neck or upper back pain

A cough or breathing problem, and maybe a hoarse voice

Emergency symptoms are like those of a cerebral event, but are more severe. If you are having the above symptoms with intensity, see your doctor for early diagnosis.

Diagnosis:

This medical problem just might be found during a check-up you are having. A lot of times x-rays for something else may see it, or other tests you are having such as an ultrasound or CT scan for a different reason. Treatments before problems begin can be done before an emergency event.

Sleeping Issues Related to Diabetes

can relate to your diabetes. How can that be possible you wonder? Well compared with nondiabetics, we may experience excessive daytime sleepiness. And if there is any type of neuropathy, there is usually leg pains or bad sensations that cause insomnia.

In brittle diabetics, (those diabetics that are very hard to control), sleeping is difficult at nighttime because of the rapid changes in blood glucose levels. This causes a lot of anxiety much of the time, and especially at night, preventing you from getting your needed rest. Some sleeping problems with diabetes could relate with obesity, such as sleep apnea. Trouble breathing during sleep, goes together with impaired glucose tolerance, and the insulin resistance you may have. A common type of sleep apnea, known as obstructive sleep apnea, is a sleep disordered breathing. There is also another type called central-type apnea where periodic breathing problems have been experienced in people with autonomic diabetic neuropathy.

Peripheral neuropathy also is another common source for sleeping troubles in diabetics. Restless legs syndrome can cause many disturbances, which contribute to sleeplessness in some people with diabetes.

How do you manage sleeping problems and your diabetes? First of all recognize what problems you have concerning this issue. Do you snore loudly? Is falling asleep hard for you? Do you suddenly gasp for air or have lapses in breathing?

Do you have painful neuropathies, or frozen shoulder with a lot of pain? Once you have been evaluated for these problems with your doctor, what will you do to get some needed rest? There are several things to be done once the real issues are discovered.

For obstructive sleep apnea, weight loss helps to relieve obesity related problems. Also the identifications of anatomic and functional airway problems and treatment help. Continuous airway pressure and some physical activity before bedtime hours has been known to help.

Restless Leg Syndrome

If you have **restless leg syndrome problems,** dopamine agonist medications, and benzodiazepines have been prescribed by doctors to help this problem.

For your **peripheral neuropathies**, there should be great focus by your doctor on controlling pains associated with that problem.

Antidepressants such as Zoloft for instance work to help you sleep, and feel better the next day, being able to live life.

Behavioral management helps a lot of people in the management of insomnia. Relaxation therapies help, and I myself, find that reading my books until very sleepy helps tremendously. Reading until you are almost asleep on the book will work well for many people. This is a great behavioral strategy. Set a time to get to bed, read a book, and sleep will eventually come.

Healthier Recipes for People with Diabetes

I have accumulated several recipes over the years that are "diabetic friendly." Enjoy them!

Butternut Squash Smashed Potatoes

1 pound (about 3 medium) yellow-flesh potatoes, cut into 3/4 inch chunks
1 small butternut squash (about 1 pound), peeled and cut into 1-inch chunks
1 tsp. kosher salt
3 tbsp butter, divided
8-10 fresh sage leaves, cut into 1/4 inch strips
1/2 cup 1 percent milk
freshly ground black pepper to taste

In a 3-quart saucepan, cover potatoes and squash with water. Add 1 tsp. salt. Bring to a boil over high high. Reduce heat, cover and cook until tender, 12-15 minutes. Meanwhile. add tablespoons of the butter and the sage to a small skillet or saucepan over medium heat. Tilting the pan and watching it closely, cook about 3 minutes, until butter foams and begins to brown. Keep warm.

Thoroughly drain potatoes and squash. Return to pan and shake 1 to 2 minutes over low heat. Roughly mash with hand masher, leaving mixture chunky. Over low heat, gently mix the remaining tablespoon of butter and enough milk to reach a desired consistency. Season with salt and pepper. Spoon into a serving bowl and drizzle with the brown butter and sage sauce. Serving size is 1 cup each,

Blueberry Dream Muffins

2 cups all-purpose flour
2 tsps baking powder
1/2 cup granulated sugar
1 large egg, lightly beaten
1 cup Rice Dream rice beverage, original (unenriched)
1/4 cup vegetable oil

1 tbsp lemon zest
1 cup frozen blueberries

Preheat oven to 375.
Combine flour, baking powder, and sugar in mixing bowl.
In a separate bowl, combine egg, Rice Dream, vegetable oil and lemon zest.
Pour liquid ingredients into flour mixture. Mix ingredients lightly until moistened, do not overmix.

Gently fold blueberries into batter.
Lightly spray 12 muffin tins with nonstick cooking spray.

Spoon batter into muffin tins.

Bake for 25 minutes or until toothpick comes out clean. Serving size is 1 muffin.

Tips
An alternative to spraying muffin tin with cooking spray is to line tins with muffin paper.
Freeze extra muffins to microwave for 30 seconds to serve later.

Apple Muffin Recipe

12 muffin papers
2 eggs
1 cup sugar
1/2 cup canola oil
1/4 cup water
1 tbsp vanilla
1-1/2 cups all purpose white flour
1 tsp baking soda
1-1/2 tsps cinnamon
1-1/2 cups raw apple, peeled and cut into small pieces

Preheat oven to 400 and place muffin papers in muffin pan.

Beat eggs in a large bowl. Add sugar, oil and water; mix well. Add vanilla.

In a separate bowl, combine flour, baking soda and 1 teaspoon cinnamon.

Stir flour mixture into egg mixture. Batter will be lumpy. Fold in apple pieces.

Fill muffin cups 3/4 full. Mix remaining 1/2 teaspoon cinnamon with 1 teaspoon sugar. Sprinkle on top of muffins.

Bake for 20 minutes or until lightly browned.

Tips: Try freezing leftover muffins and reheating in the microwave for 30 to 60 seconds for a quick snack.

Sugar can be replaced with Splenda sugar free sweetener. Be aware muffins will not rise as high and may cook 3 to 5 times faster than the recipes expected baking time. Serving size is 1 muffin.

Apple Onion Omelet

Recipe submitted by DaVita dietitian Brenda from Washington.

Portions: 2

Serving size: 1/2 omelet

Ingredients

* 3 eggs
* 1/4 cup liquid non-dairy creamer
* 1 tablespoon water
* freshly ground black pepper to taste
* 1 tablespoon butter or margarine
* 3/4 cup onion, sliced very thin (Walla Walla sweet onion recommend)
* 1 large semi-sweet apple, peeled, cored, and thinly sliced (Jonagold, Gala or McIntosh recommended)
* 2 tablespoons grated cheddar cheese

Preparation

1. Preheat oven to 400° F.

2. Beat eggs with nondairy creamer, water and ground pepper in a small bowl; set aside.

3. Over medium heat, melt butter or margarine in small, ovenproof skillet.

4. Add onion and apple to the skillet and sauté until onion becomes translucent, about 5 to 6 minutes.

5. Spread out the onion and apple mixture evenly in the skillet and sprinkle cheddar cheese over it.

6. Pour egg mixture evenly into the skillet and cook over medium heat until the edges begin to set. Transfer skillet to the oven and bake until the center is firmly set, approximately 10 to 12 minutes.

7. Cut omelet in half and slide each half onto an individual plate. Serve immediately. Serving size is 1 omelet each.

Chicken Vegetable Linguine

1 pound boneless, skinless chicken breasts
3 tbsps extra virgin olive oil
1/2 package (8 ounces) linguine
3/4 cup broccoli
3/4 cup cauliflower
3/4 cup baby carrots
16 grape tomatoes
2 tbsps lemon juice
3/4 tsp Mrs. Dash

Cut up chicken into small strips.

Heat pan on medium heat with 2 tbsps extra virgin olive oil.

Add chicken to pan and cook until done.

Cook 1/2 package of linguine according to package directions.
Cut up broccoli and cauliflower to bite-size pieces.

When chicken is cooked, add broccoli, cauliflower, carrots, tomatoes and lemon juice, cover and cook for 3 minutes.

Add drained pasta to pan and then add 1 tablespoon extra virgin olive oil and stir.

Add Mrs. Dash, stir and simmer on low for 5 minutes. Serving size is 1 cup.

Fresh Vegetable Marinade

3 cups raw broccoli florets
3 cups cauliflower broken into florets
2 cups mushroom, sliced
1 cup green pepper, sliced
1 cup celery, sliced
1/2 cup sugar
2 tsps dry mustard
1/2 tsp salt
1/2 cup vinegar
1 cup olive oil
1/2 cup onion, finely chopped
1 tbsp poppy seeds

Cut broccoli and cauliflower into bite-sized pieces. Combine with mushrooms, pepper and celery.

In a separate bowl, combine remaining ingredients to make marinade. Mix well and pour over vegetables. Refrigerate at least 3 hours before serving.

Use a slotted spoon and remove vegetables from marinade before serving. Nutrition per serving 3/4 cup each:

Cookie Salad

5.1 ounce package Jell-O Instant Vanilla Pudding Mix
1 cup liquid non-dairy coffee creamer
12-ounce tub of Cool Whip dessert topping
20 ounce can pineapple tidbits, packed in juice, drained
2 of 10.5-ounce cans light mandarin oranges, drained
12-ounce box vanilla wafers

In large bowl, combine instant vanilla pudding and creamer. Mix well. Fold Cool Whip into pudding.

Fold fruit into pudding mixture.

Place vanilla wafers in large zip-lock bag and crush with a rolling pin or mallet.

Fold 3/4 of the crushed wafers into the pudding mixture.

Top pudding with remaining wafer crumbs.

Refrigerate overnight for 2 to 3 hours before serving. Serving size is ½ cup each.

Anadama Bread

1 package (1/4 oz) active dry yeast
1 tbsp sugar
1 1/4 cups warm water (110F in temperature)
2 tbsp lite buttery spread, melted (such as Promise, Activ)
2 tbsp dark molasses

1 tsp salt
3 1/2 cups bread flour
1 cup yellow cornmeal
Vegetable oil to grease the bowl and pans
Egg Wash
1 egg
2 tbsp water

In a large mixing bowl, combine the yeast, sugar, and 1/4 cup of the water. Set aside for 10 minutes until the yeast becomes active and looks frothy.

Add the melted butter, molasses, salt, flour, and cornmeal. Add in the remaining water, mixing well with a wooden spoon. Use enough water to form a soft but not overly sticky dough. (You may need extra water). Turn out the dough on a lightly floured surface. Knead by hand for about 15 minutes, until dough is elastic and smooth.

Lightly oil a large bowl. Shape the dough into a large ball. Add the dough to the bowl and turn over so the entire ball has a film of oil on the surface. Cover with plastic wrap and then a tea towel, and place in a draft-free spot. Let the dough double in volume, about 1 hour.
Lightly oil two (9 1/2-by 5-inch) loaf pans. Turn the dough onto a lightly floured surface and cut in half. Shape each half into a loaf and place in the pans. Cover with plastic wrap, then a tea towel, and place in a draft-free spot for 30 minutes.

Preheat the oven to 350. Combine the egg and water and brush the top of the loaves with a pastry brush. Bake the loaves for 1 hour until golden brown. Remove from the oven and let cool for 10 minutes in the pans. Turn the loaves out and let them cool completely on a rack before slicing. Serving size is 1 slice.

Whole Wheat Pumpkin Bread

Nonstick cooking spray
1/2 cup all-purpose flour
1/2 cup whole wheat flour
1/2 tsp salt
1 cup Splenda No Calorie Sweetener
1 tsp baking soda
1 cup pumpkin puree
1/2 cup canola oil
1 whole egg
1 egg white
1/3 cup water
1/4 tsp nutmeg
1/4 tsp cinnamon
1/4 tsp allspice

Preheat oven to 350. Spray a 9x5x3 loaf pan with nonstick cooking spray. In a large mixing bowl, combine all ingredients in the order listed, stirring after each addition. Stir only enough to combine ingredients into a smooth batter. Pour into prepared pan. Bake 45-50 minutes, until a cake tester inserted into the center of the loaf comes out clean. Serving slice is 1 slice each.

Chicken Tortilla Soup
2 14 ounce cans reduced-sodium chicken broth
1 14-1/2 ounce can no-salt added stewed tomatoes
2 cups chopped cooked chicken breast
2 cups frozen peppers and onions
3 cloves garlic, minced
1/4 to 1/2 teaspoon crushed red pepper
4 of 6 inch corn tortillas

In a 3 and 1/2 quart slow cooker, combine chicken broth, undrained tomatoes, chicken, frozen vegetables, garlic, and crushed red pepper. Cover and cook on low heat setting for 6 to 7 hours or on high heat setting for 3 to 3 and 1/2 hours.

Before serving, preheat oven to 350. Cut tortillas into 1/2 inch-wide strips. Place in a single layer on a baking sheet. Bake for 10-12 minutes or until golden brown and crisp. Let cool on baking sheet.

To serve, ladle soup into bowls. Sprinkle with tortilla strips and, if desired, light sour cream, sliced jalapeno peppers, and additional crushed pepper. Serving size is 1 generous cup.

Green Garden Minestrone

1 tbsp olive oil
1 cup sliced celery
2/3 cup finely chopped leek
6 green onions, sliced
1 clove garlic, finely chopped
4 cups reduced-sodium chicken broth or stock
2 cups water
1 1/2 cups sliced fresh green beans and/or fresh or frozen green beans
1/2 cup dried tiny shell pasta
1/4 tsp ground black pepper
1 pound asparagus spears, trimmed and thinly sliced, or 8 ounces baby zucchini, sliced
6 cups fresh baby spinach leaves coarsely chopped, or 1 1/2 cups finely shredded green cabbage
1/4 cup snipped fresh basil
2 ounces thinly shaved Parmesan cheese

In a 4-quart Dutch oven, heat oil over medium heat. Add celery, leek, green onions, and garlic; cook until crisp-tender, stirring occasionally. Add broth, the water, green beans, pasta, and pepper.

Heat to boiling; reduce heat. Simmer, uncovered, for 10 minutes. Stir in the asparagus and spinach; simmer for 2 to 3 minutes more or until pasta and vegetables are tender. Stir in basil.

To serve, if desired, top individual servings with Parmesan cheese. Serving size is 1 ½ cups.

Vegetarian Chili

Nonstick cooking spray
1 tsp canola oil
1 cup chopped onion
1 cup chopped green sweet pepper
2 cloves garlic, minced, or 1 tsp bottle minced garlic
1 14 and 1/2 ounce can no-salt added diced tomatoes or stewed tomatoes, undrained
1 oz. can no-salt-added tomato sauce
1 cup water
4 1/2 tsps chili powder
1 tsp garlic-herb-salt-free seasoning blend
1 tsp ground cumin
1/8 tsp salt
1 15-16 ounce can kidney beans, rinsed and drained
1 cup frozen mixed vegetables
1/4 cup light dairy sour cream (optional)
Coarsely snipped fresh cilantro (optional)

Lightly coat an unheated large saucepan or Dutch oven with nonstick cooking spray. Preheat over medium high heat.

Add oil; swirl to coat the bottom of the pan. Add onion, sweet pepper, and garlic to hot oil; cook for 8-10 minutes or until pepper is tender, stirring often. If necessary, reduce heat to prevent burning.

Add tomatoes, tomato sauce, the water, 4 1/2 teaspoons chili powder, seasoning blend, cumin, and salt. Bring to boiling. reduce heat. Cover, simmer for 15 minutes.

Stir in kidney beans and mixed vegetables. Return to boiling, reduce heat. Simmer, uncovered, about 10 minutes more or until vegetables are tender.

If desired, top each serving with sour cream. Serving size is 1 cup.

Sausage and Pepper Medley

4 uncooked turkey Italian sausage links
1 tbsp olive oil
2 cloves garlic
4 medium sweet peppers, cut into thin strips
1 large onion, thinly sliced and separated into rings
1 14 1/2-ounce can no-salt-added diced tomatoes, undrained
1 1/2 teaspoons dried Italian seasoning-crushed

In a nonstick skillet, brown sausage links over medium heat. Cover and cook on medium-low about 10 minutes or until juices run clear. Thinly bias slice sausage links. Set aside.

Add olive oil and garlic to the skillet, increase heat to medium. Cook garlic for 30 seconds. Add peppers and onion; cook about 5 minutes.

Add the remaining ingredients. Bring to boiling; reduce heat. Simmer, uncovered, for 5 minutes. If desired, sprinkle with Parmesan cheese. Serving size is 1 sausage link and 1 cup of the vegetables.

Salmon and Vegetables

2 of a 4-ounce fresh or frozen skinless salmon fillets
10 ounces fresh asparagus spears, trimmed
6 ounces tiny new potatoes, cut into 1-inch pieces
2 tbsps white or regular balsamic vinegar
1 tsp cooking oil
1 tsp snipped fresh dill or 1/2 tsp dried dill
1/4 tsp salt
1/8 tsp ground black pepper
Fresh dill is optional.

Thaw salmon, if frozen. Rinse salmon and pat with paper towels. Arrange salmon in a microwave safe 2-quart square baking dish.

Arrange asparagus and potatoes around salmon. In a small bowl, combine balsamic vinegar, oil, snipped or dried dill, salt, and pepper. Drizzle over salmon and vegetables.

Cover with vented plastic wrap. Microwave on 100 percent power (high) for 10 to 12 minutes or until fish flakes easily when tested with a fork and vegetables are tender, turning dish once halfway through cooking if necessary. If desired, garnish individual servings. Serving size is about 1 cup.

Greek Feta Chicken

4 oz uncooked orzo
4 oz skinless boneless chicken breasts
2 tsp ground oregano
1/2 tsp salt
1/4 tsp fresh ground black pepper
1/8 tsp ground red pepper
1 tbsp olive oil, divided
1 small red pepper, sliced into strips
1 small green pepper, sliced into strips
2 tsp bottled minced garlic

1 and 1/2 tbsp fresh lemon juice
1 oz crumbled feta cheese

Cook the orzo according to package directions (but without added salt or fat). While the orzo cooks, sprinkle the chicken breasts with oregano, salt, pepper, and ground red pepper.

Heat 2 tsp. of the oil in a large nonstick skillet over medium-high heat. Add the chicken breasts and cook on both sides for about 4 to 5 minutes until no longer pink. Remove the chicken from the skillet.
Drain orzo and keep warm.

Lower the heat to medium and add remaining oil. Saute the peppers for 3 minutes. Add the garlic and saute for 1 minute more. Add the lemon juice and cook for 1 minute. Add back the chicken breasts to the skillet. Top with feta cheese, cover and cook 1 minute until cheese slightly melts. Serve over cooked orzo. Serving size is 1 chicken breast with 1 cup orzo.

Angel Strawberry Delight

1 package Angel Food Cake mix

One 8-ounce package of light or regular cream cheese, softened
1/2 cup strawberry preserves or low-sugar strawberry preserves
One 8-ounce container non-dairy whipped topping

Bake angel food cake according to package directions. Cool to room temperature.

Beat cream cheese and strawberry preserves until smooth.

Slice angel food cake into three even horizontal layers.

Spread cream cheese mixture between layers and reassemble.

Frost cake using nondairy whipped topping.
Keep refrigerated until ready to serve. Serving size is ¼ of cake,

Easy Apple Oatmeal Crisp

1 cup oatmeal (not quick cooking)
3/4 cup brown sugar
1/2 cup all-purpose white flour
1 tsp cinnamon
1/2 cup butter
5 Granny Smith apples, peeled, cored, sliced

Preheat oven to 350.

In a bowl, mix oatmeal, brown sugar, flour and cinnamon.

Cut butter into oatmeal mixture with a pastry cutter until well blended.
Place sliced apples in 9 x 9 baking pan. Sprinkle oatmeal mixture over
apples. Bake for 30-35 minutes. Serving size is about ⅔ cups.

Blueberry Bread Pudding

Nonstick cooking spray
1 1/2 cups fresh blueberries
3 cups reduced-fat milk (2 percent)
1/3 cup packed light brown sugar
1/2 tsp ground cinnamon
1/4 tsp ground ginger
1/2 cup white cornmeal

Preheat oven to 350. Lightly coat six 6 ounce ramekins with non-stick
cooking spray; set ramekins in a shallow baking pan and set aside.

In a large saucepan, warm milk over medium heat. Stir in brown sugar, cinnamon, and ginger. Cook and stir until ginger is dissolved.
 Slowly stir or whisk in cornmeal. Cook and stir over medium heat until bubbly. Reduce heat to medium-low; cook and stir for 3 minutes more. Mixture will thicken.

Spoon half of the cornmeal mixture evenly into prepared ramekins. Top with blueberries. Spoon remaining cornmeal mixture over blueberries. Bake for 40 to 50 minutes or until edges are bubbly. Cool on a wire rack for 20 to 30 minutes. Serve warm. Serving is about ⅔ cups.

French Toast Recipe Santa Fe Style

4 slices white bread, 3/4" thick
4 eggs or 1 cup egg substitute
1-1/4 cup nondairy creamer
2 tbsps canola oil

Preheat oven to 400.
Trim crust and cut bread in half diagonally

Beat egg slightly and add to nondairy creamer
Pour oil into a skillet and heat

Dip bread into egg mixture. Fry in oil until brown on both sides. Place browned toast pieces on a hot baking sheet. Cook for 4 minutes in the oven to puff the toast.

Remove from oven and drain on paper towel if needed. Serve immediately with powdered sugar, syrup, or jelly. Serving size is 2 pieces.

Garlic Mashed Potatoes

First, get a large cooking pot or pan of water.
2 cups baking potatoes
2 garlic cloves peeled
1/4 cup margarine or butter
1/4 cup half and half or liquid non-dairy creamer

Peel and slice the potatoes into small pieces then add to a large pot of water. Let potatoes soak for at least 4 hours. Drain off water and repeat process. (This is called leaching, which removes some of the potassium) for kidney patients.

Add new water. Boil potatoes and garlic over medium heat until soft. Drain off cooking water.

Whip potatoes and garlic with beater, slowly adding margarine and creamer until whipped smooth. Serving size is about 1;/2 cup.

Dirty Rice

3/4 cup uncooked rice
2 tsps vegetable oil
1/2 cup onion, chopped
1/2 cup green pepper chopped
1 clove garlic, chopped
1 cup reduced sodium chicken broth
1-1/4 cups water
1/2 tsp black pepper

In a casserole or saucepan, saute rice in oil until rice is light brown, stirring frequently.

Add onion and green pepper and continue to saute until onion and pepper are tender but not browned.

Add garlic and continue cooking for 1 minute.

Add broth, water and black pepper. Cover and bring to a boil; reduce heat and simmer about 20 minutes until rice is cooked. Serving size is ⅔ cup.

Apricot Rice Pudding

1 1/3 cups water
2/3 cup long grain rice
3/4 cup evaporated skim milk
1/4 cup diced dried apricots
2 tsp Splenda
1/4 tsp cinnamon
1/4 cup sugar free, fat-free vanilla yogurt

In a saucepan with tight-fitting lid, bring the water to a boil. Slowly add the rice and bring to a boil. Lower the heat, cover, and simmer for 18 to 20 minutes, until the rice is fluffy.

Add the evaporated milk, dried apricots and Splenda. Raise the heat to medium and cook for about 5 minutes, until the mixture looks creamy. Serve ½ cup in individual bowls topped with about 1 tbsp of yogurt.

Baked Chicken
4-pound whole roasting chicken
2/3 cups parboiled rice, uncooked
1 tbsp Worcestershire Sauce
1 tbsp olive oil
1 tsp black pepper
1/2 cup green bell pepper
2 scallions, chopped
1 cup pineapple chunks, drained
1/4 cup pineapple juice

Preheat oven to 350.

Rinse chicken and remove giblets from inside cavity. Pat dry with paper towel and rub chicken with oil.

In a medium bowl combine rice, Worcestershire Sauce, olive oil, black pepper, bell pepper, scallions, pineapple and pineapple juice. Spoon mixture into cavity of chicken to stuff.

Place chicken breast side up in a roasting pan or Dutch oven. Cook uncovered for 1-1/2 hours or until internal temperature reaches 180-185. Rice stuffing should reach at least 165. Let chicken rest 10-15 minutes,

Spoon rice stuffing from chicken cavity and place on a serving platter. Cut chicken into pieces, add to platter and serve.

180-185. Rice stuffing should reach at least 165. Let chicken rest 10-15 minutes.

Spoon rice stuffing from chicken cavity and place on a serving platter. Cut chicken into pieces, add to platter and serve. Serving size is 4 ounces chicken and about ⅓ cup rice.

Baked Trout

2 pounds rainbow trout fillets
1 tbsp cooking oil or spray oil
1/2 tsp salt
1 tsp salt-free lemon pepper
1/2 tsp paprika

Preheat oven to 350.

Wash and dry fillets. Rub lightly with oil.

In a large baking dish, place the fillets skin down.

Combine seasonings in a small bowl. Sprinkle evenly over fillets.

Bake uncovered for 20 to 30 minutes or until the trout fillets flake easily with a fork.

For Grilling:

Preheat grill on high heat.
Spray or brush fillet side of the trout fillets lightly with oil. Combine seasonings in a small bowl. Sprinkle evenly over fillets.

Place directly on the grill, fillet side down. Cook for 4 minutes. Spray or brush skin lightly with oil. Turn fillets over and cook until fish flakes easily with fork, about 3 to 5 minutes. Serving size is about 3 ounces.

Cabbage Rolls

12 cabbage leaves
1 pound ground turkey
1/2 cup uncooked rice
1/4 cup onion, finely chopped
2 eggs
1/4 tsp black pepper
1/4 tsp basil
2 tsps parsley
1/4 cup water
3 ounces tomato paste
2 tbsps lemon juice
1 cup water
1/8 tsp black pepper
1 tbsp sugar

Carefully remove 12 cabbage leaves from a cabbage and wash them.
Boil a large pot of water. Add cabbage leaves and cook for 2 minutes to

soften. Drain and set leaves aside.

In a large bowl, combine ground turkey, rice, onion, eggs, pepper, basil, parsley and water.

Place 1/4 cup of the turkey mixture on the cabbage leaf and fold sides of leaf over turkey mixture.
Place rolls close together, seam side down on a baking dish.

Combine tomato paste, lemon juice, water, pepper and sugar to make a sauce. Top rolls with sauce. Cover and bake at 275 for 1-1/2 hour. Uncover and bake 30 minutes longer. Serving is 2 cabbage rolls.

Cincinnati Chili Original 5 Ways

2 tbsps oil
2 1/2 pounds ground beef
4 cups cold water
1 can (6 ounces) tomato paste
2 large onions, diced
1 1/2 tbsps vinegar
1 tsp Worcestershire sauce
2 cloves garlic, crushed
2 tbsps chili powder
5 bay leaves
2 tbsps cinnamon
1 tsp allspice
2 tsps cayenne pepper
1 1/2 tbsp unsweetened cocoa
Salt and pepper to taste
8 ounces spaghetti
2 cups shredded cheddar cheese
8 green onions, chopped
1 can (15 ounces) kidney beans, drained

Place a heavy pot over medium high heat and spray with cooking spray. Add the ground beef, onions, and garlic, stirring to break the meat into small pieces. When the beef has browned, add water and bring to a boil. Reduce to a simmer and add tomato paste, vinegar, Worcestershire sauce, chili powder, bay leaves, cinnamon, allspice, cayenne pepper, and cocoa.

Let the chili simmer for 1 1/2 to 2 hours. before serving. Cook spaghetti according to the manufacturer's directions. To serve, place the spaghetti in individual bowls. Top with chili, cheddar cheese, green onion, and kidney beans. Serving size is 9 ounces.

Braised Beef Brisket

2-1/2 pounds beef brisket, fat trimmed (3-1/2 pounds untrimmed)
2 tsps black pepper
2 tbsps canola oil
1 cup onion, diced
1/2 cup celery diced
1/2 cup carrot, diced
3 bay leaves, crumbled
1 tbsp fresh parsley, chopped
2 cups reduced sodium beef broth
2 to 3 cups water
2 tbsps balsamic vinegar

Trim fat from beef and sprinkle with black pepper.

Using a heavy pot or Dutch oven, heat oil over medium-high heat and brown meat 5 minutes on each side.
Remove meat and add onion, celery and carrots. Cook and stir 4 minutes to deglaze the pot.

Add bay leaves and parsley to vegetable mixture, and place meat on top of vegetables.

Pour broth, water and balsamic vinegar over meat to cover and heat until liquid boils.

Cover pot and cook in the oven at 350 for 1-1/2 hours. Turn meat over and cook an additional 1-1/2 hours until meat is tender enough to cut with a fork.

Remove meat from pot. Add one cup water to pan juices and stir. Strain liquid from solids. Discard vegetables and reserve broth for gravy. Serving size is about 4 ounces meat and ¼ cup gravy.

Chicken Wild Rice Soup

2 tbsps butter
1 tbsp onion minced
1/4 cup all-purpose flour
4 cups low-sodium chicken broth
1 cup wild rice, cooked
1 cup white rice, cooked
8 ounces chicken breast, cooked and chopped
1 cup carrots
1 cup Coffee Rich non-dairy creamer
1 tbsp almonds slivered
parsley or chives, minced

Melt butter in a saucepan; add onion and saute until tender.
Blend in flour; gradually add chicken broth

Cook over medium heat, stirring constantly, until mixture thickens slightly.

Stir in both wild and white rice, chicken, and carrots. Simmer 5 minutes.

Blend in nondairy creamer. Heat to serving temperature.
Add almonds: garnish with minced parsley or chives before serving.
Serving size is about 1 cup.

Barbecue Meatballs

3 pounds ground beef
2 large eggs beaten
1/2 cup skim milk or nondairy milk substitute
1 cup dry oatmeal flakes (Quaker quick cooking oats)
1/2 cup onions, diced
1 tbsp dried thyme
1 tsp dried oregano
1/2 tsp pepper
1 cup barbecue sauce (look for the lower sodium brands)

Preheat oven to 375.

Combine all ingredients, except barbecue sauce and water, in a large bowl
and mix together.

Roll into 1" balls and place on a baking sheet

Bake for 10-15 minutes, until meatballs are cooked through.

Combine barbecue sauce and water in a warming dish or crock pot on low
temperature setting. Add meatballs and stir. Cover until ready to serve.
Serving size is 2 meatballs.

Versatile Saucy Meatballs

1/3 cup water
1/4 cup bulgur

1 egg

1 tsp dried Italian seasoning, chili powder, or salt-free Cajun seasoning

1/4 tsp salt

1/8 tsp ground black pepper

1 pound uncooked ground turkey or extra-lean ground beef (90 percent lean or higher)

1 of a 14 1/2 ounce can Italian-, Mexican-, or Cajun-style stewed tomatoes, undrained, cut up

2 cups hot cooked spaghetti squash (optional)

2 tbsps small fresh basil or cilantro leaves or thinly sliced green onion

In a large microwave-safe bowl, combine the water and bulgur. Microwave on 100 percent power (high) for 1 minute; do not drain. Cool slightly.

Stir egg, desired seasoning, salt, and pepper into bulgur mixture. Add ground turkey or beef; mix well. Shape into 24 meatballs. Place in a microwave-safe 2-quart square baking dish. Cover with vented plastic wrap. Microwave on 100 percent power (high) for 4 minutes, rearranging once; drain off liquid.

Pour undrained stewed tomatoes over meatballs. Cover with vented plastic wrap. Microwave on 100 percent power (high) for 1 to 3 minutes or until meatballs are no longer pink in centers (165 F). If desired, serve meatballs over spaghetti squash. Sprinkle with basil, cilantro, or green onion. Serving size is 6 meatballs.

Beef and Veggie Stir Fry

1/4 cup reduced sodium beef broth

2 tbsps reduced sodium soy sauce

1 tbsp grated fresh ginger, or 1 tsp ground ginger

1 clove garlic, finely chopped

1/2 tsp finely grated orange peel

1 tbsp vegetable oil

1 top round steak (about 12 ounces) trimmed and cut into thin strips.

1 medium green or red bell pepper cut into strips (about 1 cup)

1 cup thinly sliced carrot

1 cup thinly sliced celery

1/2 cup thinly sliced green onion (including tops)

1/2 cup thinly sliced mushrooms

2 cups bean sprouts (optional)

In a small bowl, combine broth, soy sauce, ginger, garlic, and orange peel. Mix well; set aside.

In a wok or large nonstick skillet, heat oil over high heat. Add beef and stir-fry just until no longer pink, about 3 minutes. Using a slotted spoon, place beef on a plate.

Add bell pepper, carrot, celery, green onion, and mushrooms to wok. Stir in broth mixture. Stir-fry until vegetables are crisp-tender, about 4 minutes.

Stir in bean sprouts and beef; stir-fry for 2 minutes. Place on serving plates; serve over rice or chinese noodles. Serving size is 1 cup.

Barbecue Ranch Wraps

2 tbsps bottled reduced-fat-ranch salad dressing

1 tbsps light mayonnaise or salad dressing

2 cups packaged shredded broccoli (broccoli slaw mix)

4 8-inch whole grain flour tortillas

2 tbsps bottle barbecue sauce

8 ounces cooked chicken breast or turkey breast, shredded

In a medium bowl, combine ranch dressing and mayonnaise; stir in shredded broccoli.

Spread tortillas with barbecue sauce. Top with chicken.
Top with broccoli mixture. Roll up tortillas; slice in half if desired, and
serve. Serving size is 1 wrap each.

Caraway Coleslaw

3 tbsps cider vinegar
3/4 tsp caraway seeds, crushed
1/2 tsp dry mustard
1/2 tsp prepared horseradish
1/4 tsp salt
1/4 tsp ground black pepper
1 of a 6-ounce carton plain low-fat yogurt
3 tbsps light dairy sour cream
2 tsps sugar or sugar substitute equivalent to 2 teaspoons sugar
1 of a 16-ounce package shredded cabbage with carrot (coleslaw mix)

In a small bowl, combine vinegar and caraway seeds. Cover and let stand
for 15 minutes; strain through a fine-mesh strainer into a large bowl.
Discard seeds. Add mustard, horseradish, salt, and pepper to strained
mixture; whisk until well mixed.

Whisk in yogurt, sour cream, and sugar. Add coleslaw mix; gently stir to
coat. Cover and chill for 1 to 8 hours before serving (the volume will
decrease as the salad chills). Stir before serving.

If you use sugar substitutes choose from Splenda granular, Equal spoonful
or packets, or Sweet'N Low bulk or packets. Follow package directions to
use product amount equivalent to 2 teaspoons sugar. Serving is ⅔ cup
each.

Popcorn Balls
1/2 cup butter

40 large marshmallows
1/2 tsp vanilla extract
16 cups unsalted popcorn, popped
1/2 tsp red or green food coloring (optional)

Place butter and marshmallows in a saucepan and cook over low heat, stirring until melted. Remove from heat and stir in vanilla and optional food coloring.

Place popped popcorn in a large bowl. Pour in marshmallow and stir.

To make these into balls, grease hands with butter and form popcorn balls about the size of a baseball. Place on wax paper to cool. Serve or store wrapped in plastic wrap. Serving size is 1 ball.

Cheesy Baked Ziti

8 ounces ziti pasta
8 ounces lean ground beef
1 cup shredded part-skim mozzarella cheese
1/4 cup fresh parsley
2 cups tomato sauce
1 tsp oregano
1/2 tsp basil
1/2 tsp garlic powder
1/4 tsp black pepper
1/8 tsp hot red pepper flakes
2 tsps parmesan cheese grated

Cook pasta according to package directions. Drain.
While pasta is cooking, prepare beef. In a large nonstick skillet, cook beef over medium heat, stirring until browned, about 5 minutes. Drain grease. Preheat oven to 375. In a large bowl, combine beef, pasta, mozzarella, ricotta, and parsley flakes. Mix well.

In a small bowl, combine tomato sauce, oregano, basil, garlic powder, black pepper, and red pepper flakes. Mix well. Pour 1/4 cup tomato sauce into an 8-inch square baking pan. Spread over bottom of pan. Spread pasta mixture over sauce. Top with remaining tomato sauce and Parmesan.

Bake pasta until heated through and sauce bubbles, about 30-35 minutes. Serve immediately.

Cheesy Vegetable Casserole

1 1/2 cups water
4 medium white or yellow potatoes, peeled and sliced 1/2-inch thick
1 cup bite-size raw cauliflower florets
1 cup bite-size raw broccoli florets
4 medium carrots, peeled and sliced into 1/4-inch coins
1 medium onion, chopped
2 cups frozen, cut green beans
Nonstick cooking spray
1 can (10 3/4 ounces) reduced-fat, reduced-sodium cream of chicken soup
1/2 cup skim milk
1 cup shredded reduced-fat Cheddar cheese

Bring water to a boil in a large pot over high heat. Add the potatoes and cook, covered, for 5 minutes.

Add the cauliflower, broccoli, carrots, onion, and frozen green beans. Return water to a boil, cover, and cook 10 to 12 minutes until vegetables are tender. Drain.
Spray a 2-quart baking dish with cooking spray. Add cooked vegetables. Combine the canned soup and milk. Pour soup mixture over the vegetables, mixing gently.

Preheat oven to 350°F. Cover and bake casserole for 20 to 25 minutes.

Uncover and sprinkle with cheese. Bake 3 to 4 minutes longer, until cheese melts. Serving size is ½ cup each.

Macaroni and Cheese

12 ounces elbow macaroni
2 tsps vegetable oil divided
1 medium red onion, chopped about 1 cup
1/2 cup thin red bell pepper strips
1/4 cup chopped green onion
1/2 cup sliced mushrooms
1 cup low-fat ricotta cheese
1/2 cup tomato sauce
1/3 cup shredded reduced fat cheddar cheese, divided

Cook macaroni according to your package directions.
While macaroni is cooking, in a large nonstick skillet, heat 1 tsp of oil over medium heat. Add red onion, bell pepper, and green onion; saute until vegetables begin to soften, about 4 minutes. Add remaining oil and mushrooms; saute for 4 minutes. Remove from heat; set aside.

Preheat broiler. Drain macaroni; return to pan. Add vegetable mixture, ricotta cheese, tomato sauce, and 3 tbsps of cheddar. Mix well. Heat over low heat until heated through, about 5 minutes.

Transfer mixture to a shallow baking dish. Sprinkle remaining cheddar over top. Broil 4 inches from heat until browned, about 3-5 minutes. Serve immediately. Serving size is about 1 cup.

Banana Bread Pudding

1 medium ripe banana mashed (about 1/2 cup)
1 can(12 ounces)evaporated skim milk
1/2 cup refrigerated egg substitute

3 tbsps firmly packed light brown sugar
1 tsp almond extract
1 tsp ground cinnamon
4 cups cubed French bread
1/2 cup frozen thawed light whipped topping

Spray a medium baking dish with vegetable cooking spray.

In a large bowl, combine banana, milk, egg substitute, brown sugar, almond extract, and 1/2 tsp cinnamon. Mix well. Add bread cubes, tossing to coat. Cover and chill for 30 minutes.

Preheat oven to 350. Place banana mixture in prepared dish. Place dish in a roasting pan filled with enough boiling water to come halfway up sides of dish.

Bake bread pudding until center is firm and a knife in the center comes out clean, about 45 minutes. Place on a wire rack and cool for 10 minutes. Top with whipped topping. Sprinkle with remaining cinnamon.
Serving size is about ⅔ cup.

Chicken Roll-Ups

4 flour tortillas or Mandarin pancakes
2 tsps vegetable oil
4 skinless, boneless chicken breast halves, (4 ounces each), cut into thin strips
1/2 medium red bell pepper, thinly sliced (about 1/2 cup)
2 cloves garlic, minced
1/2 cup hoisin sauce
2 tsps Chinese or regular mustard
1 tsp hot sesame oil
4 medium green onions, sliced
1/4 cup chopped fresh cilantro

Preheat oven to 250. Wrap tortillas together in foil. Place tortillas in oven to warm.

While tortillas are warming, in a large nonstick wok or skillet, heat oil over medium heat. Add chicken, pepper, and garlic. Stir-fry until chicken is no longer pink, about 10 minutes. Add hoisin sauce, mustard, and sesame oil. Cook, stirring until heated through, about 2 minutes.

Spoon chicken mixture evenly down center of tortillas. Sprinkle green onions and cilantro over chicken. Roll up tightly. Place on plates. Serve immediately. Serving size is 1 roll-up.

Fettucine

1 pound fettuccine pasta
1 tbsp. margarine
2 cloves garlic
1 tbsp. all-purpose flour
1 1/4 cups skim milk
3 tbsps light cream cheese, softened
3/4 cup grated Parmesan cheese
2 teaspoons parsley flakes
1/2 tsp. black pepper

Cook pasta according to your package directions. Drain.
While pasta is cooking, in a medium saucepan, melt margarine over medium heat. Add garlic; cook stirring for 1 minute. Stir in flour and cook for 1 minute. Whisk in milk until blended. Cook, whisking constantly, until thickened, about 7 minutes. Stir in cream cheese, cook for 2 minutes. Stir in parmesan cheese.

Place pasta on a large serving platter. Pour sauce over pasta. Toss to coat it. Serving size is 1 cup each.

Smorgasboard Salad

12 ounces corkscrew pasta
12 ounces red potatoes, scrubbed and quartered
1/2 medium green bell pepper, sliced
1/2 medium red bell pepper, sliced
2 cooked sirloin steaks (4 ounces each), cut into 1-inch cubes
2 tbsps chopped green onion
1 cup radicchio lettuce leaves
Dressing
2 tbsps olive oil
2 tbsps fresh lemon juice
1/2 tsp salt
1/4 tsp black pepper

Cook pasta according to package directions. Drain.

Meanwhile, bring a large pot of water to a boil. Add potatoes. Cook until almost tender, about 10 minutes. Add green pepper and red pepper. Cook until vegetables are tender, about 3 minutes longer. Drain and cool slightly.

To prepare dressing, in a large bowl, combine oil, lemon juice, salt, and pepper. Mix well. Add pasta, potato mixture, steak, and green onion to bowl; toss to combine. Line a large serving bowl with lettuce leaves. Spoon salad into bowl. Serve immediately. Serving size is 1 cup.

Corn and Potato Chowder

2 cups frozen sweet corn kernels, thawed or fresh
1 medium onions, chopped
1 tbsp vegetable oil
2 cups vegetable broth
2 cups potatoes, fresh, with skin, diced

1/2 cup freshly chopped celery,sliced
1/2 tsp ground thyme
1 3/4 cup fat free milk (or fat free half and half)
1 pinch salt
1 pinch black pepper
1 cup chopped parsley, finely chopped

In a large pot, cook corn and onions 5 to 8 minutes or until soft.
Using a blender or food processor, puree 1/2 of the corn and onion
mixture and the broth. Pour mixture back into the pot.

Mix in the potatoes, celery, and thyme and bring to a boil.
Lower heat, place lid on pot, and simmer 10 to 15 minutes or until
vegetables are soft. Mix in half and half, and cook 2 to 3 minutes.
Sprinkle with salt and pepper.

When ready to serve, top with parsley or chives. Serving size is 1 cup.

Crockpot Chicken Roasted with Lemon Flavor

1 tbsp olive oil
2 cloves garlic, minced
1 tsp oregano
2 pounds chicken breasts, with bone and skin
one 13-ounce can chicken broth
3 tbsps lemon juice

Heat oil in large skillet. Add chicken breasts and brown on all sides.
Place chicken in crock pot and a can of chicken broth. Cook on low
heat setting for 6 to 8 hours. Add lemon juice during last hour of cooking.

Ideas for this recipe:

Complete the meal with a serving of rice, green beans, French bread, margarine or butter and a baked apple for dessert.

Use leftover chicken breasts in a chicken salad or sandwich for lunch the next day.

Chocolate Covered Pretzels

6 ounces semisweet chocolate chips
12 of 7 inch pretzel rods
5 tsps red and green sprinkles

Place chocolate chips in a large saucepan over low heat and stir frequently until melted and smooth; heat carefully to avoid scorching the chocolate.

Remove saucepan from heat. Hold one pretzel, coating all except 2 inches at one end; use the back of the spoon to spread the chocolate evenly. (Rewarm chocolate over low heat as needed).

Lightly sprinkle each pretzel rod with sprinkles. Carefully place coated pretzels in a pie plate, popping the uncoated end against the edge of the pie plate.

Chill coated pretzels in the freezer for 5 minutes, or until chocolate is set. Carefully remove from the pie plate and store in an airtight container at room temperature. Serving size is 1 pretzel rod.

Corn Bread

1 cup all-purpose white flour
1 cup plain cornmeal

1/4 cup sugar
2 tsps baking powder
1/2 cup liquid egg substitute
1 cup un-enriched rice milk
2 tbsps unsalted butter, melted or 2 tbsps canola oil

Preheat oven to 400.

In a bowl, combine flour, cornmeal, sugar and baking powder.
In another bowl, combine egg substitute, rice milk and melted butter.

Stir dry ingredients into wet ingredients just until moistened.
Fill greased or paper-lined muffin cups 2/3 full.
Bake for 15 to 20 minutes or until a toothpick comes out clean.
Serve warm.

www.ingramcontent.com/pod-product-compliance
Lightning Source LLC
Chambersburg PA
CBHW070652290526
45790CB00001B/283